Hypertension
in Children

Hypertension in Children

A Practical Approach

Leonard G. Feld, M.D., Ph.D.
Professor and Vice Chairman of Pediatrics and Chief, Division of Pediatric Nephrology, State University of New York at Buffalo School of Medicine and Biomedical Sciences; Director, Children's Kidney Center and Pediatric Transplantation, Children's Hospital of Buffalo, Buffalo

Foreword by
Alan B. Gruskin, M.D.
Professor and Chairman of Pediatrics, Wayne State University School of Medicine; Pediatrician in Chief, Children's Hospital of Michigan, Detroit

Butterworth-Heinemann
Boston   Oxford   Johannesburg   Melbourne   New Delhi   Singapore

Library of Congress Cataloging-in-Publication Data

Feld, Leonard G.
    Hypertension in children : a practical approach / Leonard G. Feld.
        p. cm.
    Includes bibliographical references and index.
    ISBN 0-7506-9678-8 (alk. paper)
    1. Hypertension in children--Congresses.   I. Title.
    [DNLM: 1. Hypertension--in infancy & childhood.   WG 340 F312h
1996]
RJ426.H9F45   1996
618.92'132--dc20
DNLM/DLC
for Library of Congress   96-9301
                                              CIP

British Library Cataloguing-in-Publication Data

A catalogue record for this book is available from the British Library.

The publisher offers special discounts on bulk orders of this book.

For information, please contact:
Manager of Special Sales
Butterworth–Heinemann
313 Washington Street
Newton, MA 02158–1626
Tel: 617-928-2500
Fax: 617-928-2620

For information on all medical publications available, contact our World Wide Web home page at: http://www.bh.com/med

10 9 8 7 6 5 4 3 2 1

Printed in the United States of America

For all their support and love, Barbara, Kimberly, and Mitchell

Contents

Contributing Authors

Nuel C. Celebrado, M.D.
Clinical Instructor in Pediatrics, Division of Pediatric Nephrology, Department of Pediatrics, University Medical Center at Stony Brook, Stony Brook, New York

Leonard G. Feld, M.D., Ph.D.
Professor and Vice Chairman of Pediatrics and Chief, Division of Pediatric Nephrology, State University of New York at Buffalo School of Medicine and Biomedical Sciences; Director, Children's Kidney Center and Pediatric Transplantation, Children's Hospital of Buffalo, Buffalo

Frederick Kaskel, M.D.
Associate Professor of Pediatrics, Physiology, and Biophysics and Director, Division of Pediatric Nephrology, Department of Pediatrics, State University of New York at Stony Brook School of Medicine, Stony Brook

Marva M. Moxey-Mims, M.D.
Assistant Professor of Pediatrics, George Washington University School of Medicine; Attending Pediatric Nephrologist, Department of Pediatric Nephrology, Children's National Medical Center, Washington, D.C.

James E. Springate, M.D.
Associate Professor of Pediatrics, State University of New York at Buffalo School of Medicine and Biomedical Sciences; Attending Physician, Division of Pediatric Nephrology, Department of Pediatrics, Children's Hospital of Buffalo, Buffalo

F. Bruder Stapleton, M.D.
Ford/Morgan Professor and Chair of Department of Pediatrics, University of Washington School of Medicine, Seattle

Patricia A. Veiga, M.D.
Nephrologist, Department of Pediatrics, Children's Hospital of Orange County, Orange, California

Wayne R. Waz, M.D.
Assistant Professor of Pediatrics, State University of New York at Buffalo School of Medicine and Biomedical Sciences; Director, Chronic Dialysis Program, Division of Pediatric Nephrology, Department of Pediatrics, Children's Hospital of Buffalo, Buffalo

Foreword

Hypertension, an abnormal elevation of one of the vital signs, is not a discreet disease but an expression of a disturbance in integrative physiology. Its origin is multifaceted, and left untreated, the disease eventually involves the kidneys, heart, eye, or brain. It also accelerates any underlying atherosclerotic disease and shortens one's expected life span. Because hypertension is not organ oriented, it has not been viewed as an independent medical subspecialty but as a discipline that has fascinated and involved clinical and basic scientists, epidemiologists, public health experts, and pharmacologists.

With each succeeding decade since my first exposure to childhood hypertension more than 30 years ago, its importance as a pediatric discipline has continued to evolve and grow. The plethora of new diagnostic approaches and technologies, as well as new classes of drugs, has created confusion but simultaneously improved the quality of life for hypertensive children. Childhood hypertension has been progressively delineated as an important topic in pediatrics and is currently viewed as an independent pediatric discipline.

The importance of hypertension requires that all pediatric health care providers become knowledgeable about its impact on children. The ever-increasing body of information on the various aspects of hypertension supports the need to prioritize, focus, and organize the information that pertains to children in a useable and practical format. This text successfully sifts through the available data and provides essential background information, as well as pragmatic approaches to diagnosis and treatment, in a concise and helpful fashion. The beneficiaries of this effort will be both practitioners and children, as it makes the subject of childhood hypertension readily understandable and the care of affected children rational and cost-effective.

Alan B. Gruskin, M.D.

Preface

Almost 20 years have passed since the first *Report of the Task Force on Blood Pressure Control in Children.* This book is intended to serve as a detailed guide for pediatricians, family practitioners, and other health care providers on the methods for measuring blood pressure in infants and children, the definitions and classification of hypertension, the approach to evaluating the child with suspected hypertension, and the therapeutic options in acute and nonemergent situations. The reader should be aware that detailed descriptions of the pathophysiology of hypertension are not discussed.

In each chapter there are numerous tables and figures to illustrate key points. It is always difficult to provide precise dosing recommendations for the use of antihypertensive drugs in infants and children. As with most medications given to children, there have been limited pharmacokinetic and therapeutic trials. Our recommendations are based on our clinical experience and on the current literature. Therefore, *it always better to give less, and it is always easier to give more.* The final chapter provides discussions of the most common referrals for hypertension in our practice and answers to the most frequently asked questions from primary care physicians.

Leonard G. Feld, M.D., Ph.D.

Acknowledgments

For over 20 years, I have devoted a significant portion of my career to basic science research and to the clinical practice of treating hypertension. I would like to thank Dr. Judith B. Van Liew and the late Dr. John W. Boylan for providing me the "bench" and friendship for developing my career in the pathophysiology of hypertension. With the passing of Dr. Boylan and retirement of Dr. Van Liew, the lab will never be the same—there will always be a void.

The academic physician only succeeds with the support of his or her family. My parents and my wife have endured the hard times and the long hours.

We learn from books and lectures, but we learn most from our patients. What the books omitted is taught to us by the infants and children we treat.

I would like to thank all the staff at Butterworth-Heinemann and, in particular, Cynthia Carlson, my editor.

Leonard G. Feld, M.D., Ph.D.

"Thus 'hypertensive disease' when fully analysed is an assembly of lesions of heart and vessels having a variety of causes, one of which is arterial pressure. Cause, arterial pressure, and effects, the maladies of heart and vessels, are related quantitatively."

George Pickering, Kt. F.R.S., M.D., F.R.C.P.
Regius Professor of Medicine, University of Oxford
In *High Blood Pressure*, Grune & Stratton,
New York, 1955, p. 5.

CHAPTER 1

History of the Study of Pediatric Hypertension

F. Bruder Stapleton

> The child is father of the man
>
> —*My Heart Leaps Up*, William Wordsworth

As has been the case in many chronic conditions with childhood antecedents, arterial hypertension in children was not considered a general health concern until the last half century. Even in recent times, measurement of blood pressure has not always been an essential component of the physical examination of young children. Currently, however, pediatricians are studying the pathogenetic mechanisms of increased arterial blood pressure with the goal of developing curative or preventative strategies.

The development of our understanding of systemic blood pressure in children has resulted from the evolution of the organization of child health care, the expansion of scientific inquiry, and the dramatically increased application of new clinical technologies within the field of pediatrics. Measurement of blood pressure is now routinely performed in all pediatricians' offices and has been the subject of two comprehensive reports by the Task Force on Blood Pressure Control in Children, sponsored by the National Heart Blood and Lung Institute [1, 2]. Because the long-term adverse effects of elevated arterial blood pressure have been recognized, pediatricians have become more concerned about the early detection of hypertension and have identified groups of high-risk children. A comprehensive understanding of hypertension is now required for all pediatricians. It is only during the past several decades that this degree of clinical involvement in the treatment of hypertension in children has occurred.

1

Pre-Subspecialty Period

Early pediatric texts often provided ranges of normal blood pressure for term infants and young children [3, 4]. In these texts, pediatricians were cautioned about the vagaries of blood pressure measurement in children as well as the general inability to obtain accurate blood pressure values in children under 3 years of age. The normal systolic and diastolic blood pressure values listed for children were based on studies with small numbers of subjects. Such values were not provided for babies born prematurely, because survival of premature infants was uncommon and neonatal intensive care units did not exist.

At mid–twentieth century, pediatricians seldom focused on a subspecialty. Cardiology and endocrinology were two of the earliest well-developed pediatric subspecialities; thus, experts in pediatric hypertension initially emerged from the ranks of pediatric cardiologists and endocrinologists. Not surprisingly, in early texts, discussions of hypertension in children were largely related to the problems of coarctation of the aorta, pheochromocytoma, adrenal disorders, and acute nephritis [3, 4]. Essential hypertension, a well-recognized affliction of adults, was believed to be infrequent in children [5].

Until the 1960s, the limitations of clinical technology for the measurement of blood pressure in children significantly restricted pediatricians in their study of hypertension. The introduction of the "flush" technique for determination of systolic pressure allowed pediatricians to determine blood pressure differentials between upper and lower extremities in babies and infants [6]. Although this technique assisted in the diagnosis of coarctation of the aorta, the actual pressure values more closely reflected mean pressures, not true systolic values. When sphygmomanometry was introduced into pediatric practice, the importance of cuff width and length became apparent. Sphygmomanometric measurements were compared with intra-arterial pressures by cardiologists, and later by neonatologists during studies of premature and term infants [7, 8]. When the Doppler principle was applied to the measurement of blood pressure in 1968, its use in pediatric practice became widely accepted. It provided invaluable assistance for the emerging critical care units for children and neonates [6].

In the late 1950s and throughout the 1960s, population-based studies of childhood blood pressure were undertaken in Miami, Saint Louis, Muscatine, Iowa, and Bogalusa, Louisiana [1, 9–11]. Data from these studies provided important standards for the assessment of blood pressure in children and formed the basis for the first Task Force Report on childhood hypertension [1]. However, critical questions concerning the appropriate application of the Korotkoff sounds and the definition of what constitutes hypertension in children continued to face pediatricians.

The First (1977) and Second (1987) Reports from the Task Force on Blood Pressure Control in Children provided clarification and standardization of normal values for pediatric blood pressure [1, 2]. These useful documents provided age- and gender-appropriate standards as well as guidelines for the evaluation of children with hypertension. The first report recommended evaluation of children with blood pressures above the ninety-fifth percentile for age, while the second report proposed evaluating children above the ninetieth percentile for age. Both publications identified groups of children at risk for hypertension and reviewed available therapies for children with chronic and acute, severe hypertension. In the decade between these two reviews, the laboratory and radiologic tools available for the evaluation of hypertension had increased considerably.

Pediatric Specialization

During the 1960s, a number of pediatric subspecialties begin to evolve. Most notable for the study of hypertension were pediatric nephrology, neonatology, and pediatric radiology. Pediatric nephrology became closely linked with the study of hypertension in children. The prevailing pediatric literature discounted the possibility of essential hypertension in children, stating that 70–80% of children with hypertension had secondary forms of hypertension, and that as many as 80% of children with secondary hypertension had a renal origin for their elevated blood pressure. During the 1960s and 1970s, renovascular physiology advanced from the studies of Goldblatt in 1934 to the identification of the role of renin and angiotensin in the control of vascular tone and systemic blood pressure [12]. This identification underscored the intimate relationship of the kidney to the renin-angiotensin system and brought nephrologists into the center of the study of hypertension. As renin values were profiled with sodium excretion in adults, pediatricians naturally pursued similar studies in children, and as is often the case, found that such relationships in children were more complicated than those found in adults. In particular, neonates and infants were found to have elevated concentrations of renin and aldosterone when compared to adults or older children. These findings created considerable interest in the burgeoning field of developmental renal physiology.

During this same time period, more sensitive imaging tools were being developed to study the kidneys and the renal vasculature by pediatric radiologists. Radionuclide scans were invented that were capable of detecting pheochromocytomas and comparing both glomerular filtration and renal blood flow between the two kidneys. The development of ultrasonography provided a less invasive means of assessing renal size and excluding obstructive and mass lesions. The introduction of computed tomography provided images that were not previously available for the study of renal, adrenal, and cerebral anatomy and pathology. In addition, more sensitive angiographic techniques were developed [13]. Each of these diagnostic tools expanded the approaches available for the study of hypertension in children.

In the late 1960s and early 1970s, neonatal intensive care units were organized to provide regional resources for neonates with life-threatening disorders. The increased technology of these units dramatically improved neonatal survival for children with respiratory distress and also provided clinical laboratories in which neonatal blood pressure measurement and control were daily challenges. As a consequence of the more aggressive critical care therapies and umbilical arterial monitoring of arterial oxygenation, renal vascular thromboses with their attendant hypertension became a new clinical challenge in neonatal intensive care units [14]. As smaller babies were rescued from the problems of prematurity, the control of blood pressure in these tiny infants became the shared problem of the neonatologist and pediatric nephrologist. These scientists were later surprised to learn that intrauterine growth failure itself was a risk factor for developing hypertension later in life.

Infant nutrition has always intrigued pediatricians. When salt intake was impugned as a determinate of adult hypertension, studies were performed to assess the relationship of sodium in infant formula with childhood blood pressure. One study found that systolic blood pressure was 2.1 mm Hg higher in infants fed a "normal" sodium diet from birth compared with a similar group fed a "low" sodium diet [15]. Although the role of sodium, chloride, and even calcium in the genesis of hypertension in children was unclear, valiant efforts were waged to reduce the amount of sodium in infants' diets. In some instances, these well-intended efforts created unforeseen problems. For example, when the sodium concentration in infant formula was reduced, more episodes of dehydration and hospital admissions of infants with cystic fibrosis ensued during the summer months. Perhaps the most serious outcome of attempts to reduce the sodium content of infant formula was the chloride-deficient formula epidemic in 1979. Apparently, one formula manufacturer, while reducing the sodium concentration to approximate the sodium concentration in human milk, inadvertently depleted the formula of chloride [16]. Children who were solely dependent on this formula for nutrients and who were also dehydrated from gastroenteritis became severely alkalotic and hypokalemic. The value of sodium restriction in the prevention or treatment of many forms of hypertension remains controversial to this day.

Research Advances

The complex nature of controlling vascular tone and systemic blood pressure homeostasis has provided immense challenges to investigators and led pediatric investigators into unforeseen fields of successful inquiry. Perhaps one of the most significant opportunities for advancing the study of blood pressure control came from the development of the radioimmunoassay technique. From that time forward, hormones, peptides, and other mediators of vascular tone could be assayed from relatively small amounts of blood. During the 1970s, the kallikrein-kinin system, the prostaglandins, the natriuretic hormones, and the sympathetic nervous system were dissected, along with the renin-angiotensin system, and our understanding of vascular tone continued to expand. Concomitant with these laboratory studies, clinical investigators were examining the role of diet, obesity, exercise, race, and vascular reactivity to various stresses in children with hypertension [2, 5, 17].

Exciting new discoveries in the field of hypertension emerged in the 1980s, as molecular biological studies examined the role of intracellular calcium in the regulation of vascular smooth muscle contraction [18]. The recognition of the importance of intracellular calcium in the modulation of muscular contraction led to the introduction of calcium channel blockers as antihypertensive agents. During this time, inhibitors of angiotensin converting-enzymes also were synthesized.

During the 1980s, new mechanisms for the control of blood flow through local or regional vascular beds were discovered. Endothelin and nitric oxide became new icons with vast implications in the unraveling of the control mechanisms of peripheral vascular resistance. Receptor biology also enjoyed a strong following during this period. Again, developmental renal and vascular physiologic studies emanating from hypertension-related research provided new insights into the maturation and composition of mature biological systems, particularly related to the dopaminergic receptors [19].

The explosion of molecular biology has propelled us to new understandings of the expression of the renin gene and has clarified the basis of dexamethasone-suppressible hyperaldosteronism and the syndrome of apparent mineralocorticoid excess [20]. As the maturation of the renin-angiotensin system as been unveiled, an important role for angiotensin in organogenesis has been proposed [21].

Today's Medicine

We have learned much about hypertension in children over the past 50 years. We now recognize that essential hypertension has its origins in childhood and that it represents 80% of hypertensive adolescents [22]. Efforts to identify children at risk for essential hypertension and to prevent its occurrence are important challenges for the future. Our ability to treat hypertension has also improved dramatically since the days when the only antihypertensive drugs available for treatment of hypertensive children were reserpine, alpha-methyldopa, or guanethidine. While our armamentarium for the treatment of hypertension has vastly expanded, we remain handicapped by the knowledge that relatively few of the best antihypertensive drugs are approved for use in children. In addition, scant research data are available about the efficacy, pharmacokinetics, or long-term toxicities of antihypertensive drugs in children. Recently, we have learned about the fetopathy that is associated with maternal use of angiotensin-converting enzyme inhibition during pregnancy [23]. Assuredly, other sinister surprises from well-intended antihypertensive therapy inevitably await us.

In the 1990s, the high cost of health care is forcing physicians to re-examine current practices in order to find the most cost-efficient approaches to clinical care. Pediatricians have long been promoters of disease prevention. Nowhere in medicine is the concept of prevention or early detection with correction more cogent than in the area of hypertension. There is little debate about the adverse effect of high blood pressure on the incidence of serious cardiovascular events. It is also now apparent that hypertension accelerates the progression of established renal disease and diabetic nephropathy. As more and more children are discovered with arterial blood pressures above the ninetieth percentile, the responsibility for appropriate evaluation and effective management of these children will increasingly gravitate to the primary care pediatrician or family practitioner. The information contained in this reference text is of great importance to anyone who provides medical care for children. However, many critical answers to the essential questions about hypertension in children lay yet undiscovered.

References

1. Report of the Task Force on Blood Pressure Control in Children. Pediatrics 1977;59:797.
2. Report of the Second Task Force on Blood Pressure Control in Children—1987. Pediatrics 1987;79:1.
3. JPC Griffith, AG Mitchell (eds). Organs of Circulation. In The Diseases of Children and Infants (2nd ed). Philadelphia: Saunders, 1938;36.
4. Hughes JG. Newborn Infant. In JG Hughes (ed), Pediatrics in General Practice. New York: McGraw-Hill, 1952;34.
5. Loggie JMH. Hypertension in children and adolescents. 1. Causes and diagnostic studies. J Pediatr 1969;74:331.
6. Moss AJ. Indirect methods of blood pressure measurement. Pediatr Clin North Am 1978;25:3.
7. Park MK, Guntheroth WG. Direct blood pressure measurements in brachial and femoral arteries in children. Circulation 1970;61:231.
8. Hall RT, Oliver TK Jr. Aortic blood pressure in infants admitted to a neonatal intensive care unit. Am J Dis Child 1971;121:145.
9. Londe S, Goldring D. Blood pressure standards for normal children as determined under office conditions. Clin Pediatr (Phila) 1968;7:400.
10. Lauer RM, Clarke WR, Beaglehole R. Coronary heart disease risk factors in school children:the Muscatine study. J Pediatr 1975;86:697.

11. Voors AW, Foster TA, Frerichs RR, Webber LS. Studies of blood pressures in children ages 5–14 years in a total biracial community: the Bogalusa Heart Study. Circulation 1976;54:319.
12. Goldblatt H, Lynch J, Hanzal RF. Studies on experimental hypertension. I. The production of persistent elevation of systolic blood pressure by means of renal ischemia. J Exp Med 1934;59:347.
13. Tonkin I, Stapleton FB, Roy SR III. Digital subtraction angiography in the evaluation of renal vascular hypertension in children. Pediatrics 1988;81:350.
14. Adelman RD. Long-term follow-up of neonatal renovascular hypertension. Pediatr Nephrol 1987;1:35.
15. Hofman A, Hazebroek A, Valkenburg HA. A randomized trial of sodium intake and blood pressure in newborn infants. JAMA 1983;250:370.
16. Roy SR III, Arant BS. Hypokalemic metabolic alkalosis in normotensive infants with increased plasma renin and hyperaldosteronism: role of dietary chloride deficiency. Pediatrics 1981;67:423.
17. Murphy JK, Alpert BS, Willey ES, Somes GW. Cardiovascular reactivity to psychological stress in healthy children. Psychophysiology 1988;25:144.
18. Adelstein RS, Sellers JR. Effects of calcium on vascular smooth muscle contraction. Am J Cardiol 1987;59:4.
19. Jose PA, Martin GR, Felder, RA. Cardiovascular and Autonomic Influences on Blood Pressure. In JMH Loggie (ed), Pediatric and Adolescent Hypertension. Boston: Blackwell, 1992;33.
20. Pascoe L, Curnow KM, Slutsker L, et al. Glucocorticoid-suppressible hyperaldosteronism results from hybrid genes created by unequal crossovers between CYP11B1 and CYP11B2. Proc Natl Acad Sci U S A 1992;89:8327.
21. Gomez RA, Norwood VF. Developmental consequences of the renin-angiotensin system. Am J Kidney Dis 1995;26:409.
22. Lieberman E. Essential hypertension in children and youth: a pediatric perspective. J Pediatr 1974;85:1.
23. Sedman AB, Kershaw DV, Bunchman TE. Recognition and management of angiotensin converting enzyme inhibitor fetopathy. Pediatr Nephrol 1995;9:382.

CHAPTER 2

Measurement of Blood Pressure

Nuel C. Celebrado and Frederick Kaskel

In recent years, routine blood pressure (BP) determination in the doctor's office has been emphasized as part of the physical assessment of children. The American Academy of Pediatrics recommends annual BP determinations for children 3 years of age through adolescence during a well-child visit. It is hoped that this practice will help in the early diagnosis and management of an asymptomatic hypertensive individual before a complication such as end-organ damage occurs. BP should also be determined in children with an acute illness because an elevated BP may complicate certain diseases or be an indication of future hypertension.

The physiologic and physical factors that determine and regulate arterial BP include cardiac output (heart rate × stroke volume), peripheral vascular resistance, blood volume, and arterial compliance [1]. These factors are, in turn, affected by other forces such as the central nervous, endocrine, and renal systems. Apart from these intrinsic factors, environmental factors such as temperature, place, time of day, and season have been shown to affect actual BP levels. Because so many factors can alter BP readings, it is important that the observer not add any technical inaccuracies while doing the procedure.

Methods of Blood Pressure Determination

Auscultation Sphygmomanometry

Auscultation sphygmomanometry is the most common method used in indirect BP determination. It is accurate and easy to perform if important specific details are considered. The equipment includes a sphygmomanometer, which consists of an inflatable bladder within an unyielding cuff (Figure 2.1A), a manometer, an inflating device, and an exhaust valve. There are two types of manometers—aneroid and mercury. The aneroid manometer requires recalibration periodically. The meniscus in the reservoir of the mercury manometer must be exactly at the zero mark; if it is less, mercury must be added. A stethoscope used to listen for the Korotkoff sounds is necessary with both types of manometers.

To obtain accurate BP readings, it is essential to use a correct bladder size within the BP cuff for the patient's arm. The bladder size should not be based on the patient's age. A bladder that is too small for the patient's arm will result in an erroneously high BP, while a bladder that is too large will result in an inaccurately low BP (Figure 2.1B). Steinfeld [2] demonstrated that for infants and young children, it is necessary to use a bladder cuff in which the width equals or exceeds two-thirds the length of the extremity. Table 2.1 shows the recommended bladder dimensions based on arm size. The meniscus of the mercury should be at eye level with the examiner.

The bladder pressure cuff must be applied snugly to the bare limb, because a loosely applied cuff results in a spuriously elevated BP reading. The bladder must be inflated rapidly and deflated slowly. The examiner should first make a palpatory determination of systolic pressure in order to estimate how high to elevate the pressure in subsequent determinations [3]. Korotkoff sounds are heard better with the bell of the stethoscope placed lightly over the brachial artery pulse [4].

After rapid inflation to about 20–30 mm Hg above the estimated systolic BP, the cuff should be deflated slowly at a rate of 2–3 mm Hg per second. As the cuff pressure is being released, the examiner will hear a tapping sound. This is the Korotkoff sound; it has five phases:

- Phase I, marked by the onset of the initial tapping, is the point of systolic BP.
- Phase II is the period when a murmur is heard.
- Phase III occurs when the sounds increase in intensity and become crisper.
- As the pressure is further released, phase IV (DBP4) is signified by the onset of the muffled tap.
- Finally, the point at which sound disappears is phase V (DBP5).

The Second Task Force on Blood Pressure Control in Children recommended that phase IV be used as the measure of diastolic BP in infants and preadolescent children and phase V be used to measure BP in adolescent children and adults [5].

The examiner should note any unavoidable extraneous factors that could influence the recording. Because anxiety and apprehension can cause an elevated BP, the examiner must give the child time to relax and should approach the patient in a nonthreatening manner. It is important to

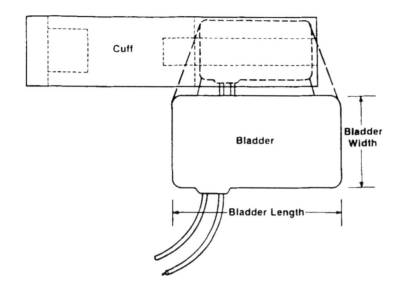

A

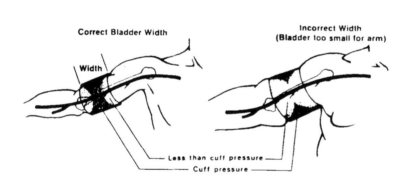

B

FIGURE 2.1. A. The bladder and cuff relationships. B. On the right, bladder width is small for the arm and the artery never has full cuff pressure applied. An erroneously high blood pressure results. On the left, the bladder width is adequate for the arm and full cuff pressure is applied to the brachial artery. (Reproduced with permission from WM Kirkendall, M Feinleib, ED Freis, et al. Recommendations for human blood pressure determination by sphygmomanometers (AHA Committee Report). Circulation 1980;62:1147. Reproduced with permission. Copyright 1980 American Heart Association.)

TABLE 2.1
Recommended Bladder Dimensions for Blood Pressure Cuff

Arm Circumference at Midpoint[a] (cm)	Cuff Name	Bladder Width (cm)	Bladder Length (cm)
5.0–7.5	Newborn	3	5
7.5–13	Infant	5	8
13–20	Child	8	13
17–26	Small adult	11	17
24–32	Adult	13	24
32–42	Large adult	17	32
42–50[b]	Thigh	20	42

[a]Midpoint of arm is defined as half the distance from the acromion to the olecranon.
[b]In large individuals (>ninety-fifth percentile for weight), the indirect blood pressure should be measured in the leg or forearm.
Source: Modified from WM Kirkendall, M Feinleib, ED Freis, AL Mark. Recommendations for human blood pressure determinations by sphygmomanometers (AHA Committee Report). Circulation 1980:62;1149.

explain the procedure to the patient, while at the same time giving reassurance. Before taking the BP, it is also important to repeat the pulse until it is stable or reproducible to avoid falsely elevated readings related to anxiety.

Flush Method

When the Korotkoff sounds are difficult to hear, examiners use the flush method of BP determination in small infants (Figure 2.2). This technique requires two observers. The pressure cuff is applied to the patient's wrist or ankle. The distal limb is drained of blood by wrapping it with an elastic bandage or a rubber glove. The pressure cuff is then inflated above the anticipated systolic pressure. The first observer unwraps the bandage and watches the blanched limb flush, while the second observer deflates and monitors the manometer. The appearance of the "flushed" color is the blood pressure reading on the manometer. Simultaneous measurements can be made in the hand and foot, but these require three observers. Readings of the flush technique have been shown to be relatively accurate. Moss and co-authors explain that the values represent the mean arterial pressure and not the systolic BP [6]. Moss also noted that the pressure at the ankle was significantly lower than at the wrist [7]. Some of the factors that could affect the reading of the end point (which is indicated by the flushed color) are peripheral vasoconstriction, marked anemia, edema, and severe hypothermia. It may also be difficult to observe the "flush" in dark-skinned individuals.

Doppler Ultrasound

Doppler ultrasound makes use of the Doppler phenomenon, which is the change in frequency of sound waves when reflected off a moving object. In

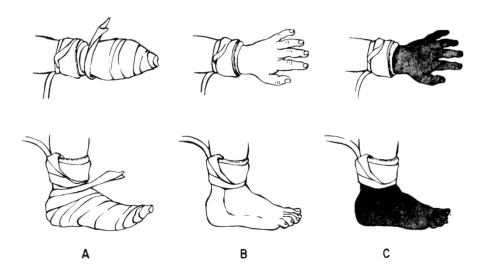

FIGURE 2.2. Flush method of blood pressure measurements. A. The cuff is applied to the wrist or ankle, and the distal portion of the extremity is wrapped snugly with an elastic bandage. B. The manometric pressure is then raised above the expected systolic blood pressure and the elastic wrapping is removed. C. The blood pressure cuff is gradually deflated until the blanched portion flushes. (Reproduced with permission from AJ Moss, FH Adams. Problems of Blood Pressure in Childhood. Springfield, IL: Charles C. Thomas, 1962.)

auscultatory sphygmomanometry, a transducer, instead of a stethoscope, is used to detect the ultrasonic signals generated by movement of arterial walls. The examiner places the transducer over the artery distal to the BP cuff. The cuff is then inflated until the vessel is occluded and no signal is audible. As the pressure is gradually decreased, the first sound generated as blood flows through the vessel is the systolic pressure. The movement of the arterial wall also generates opening and closing signals. These opening and closing signals will come closer together as they become equal to the diastolic pressure. The Doppler method has been shown to have good systolic and diastolic BP correlation with intra-arterial measurements [8–10]. It is preferred to the flush method for use in infants.

Oscillometry

The principle of oscillometry involves the detection of oscillations transmitted by arterial pulsations to a pneumatic cuff wrapped around the extremity. The Dinamap (Critikon, Tampa, FL) uses this principle to estimate arterial pressure. Colan and colleagues [11] have shown that the Dinamap provides more accurate systolic and diastolic BP values in neonates, infants, and young children than central aortic pressure measurements. Their data also documented that the Dinamap is more accurate than the Doppler instrument in measuring diastolic pressure in infants and young children.

The Dinamap is advantageous in that it requires fewer personnel for BP determinations (because it is an automatic device) and it does not use a transducer, which may be displaced by patient movement. However, the readings of arterial pressure may vary widely in a child who is crying or moving vigorously.

Random-Zero Sphygmomanometer

The random-zero sphygmomanometer has been used to reduce observer bias in clinical trials and epidemiologic studies. In principle, it is similar to the standard mercury sphygmomanometer, except for a mechanical device that is interposed between the mercury reservoir and the manometer column. This device draws variable amounts of mercury into an expandable chamber. This modification obscures the true zero level of the mercury until the end of the reading.

The procedure includes spinning a wheel that alters the height of the mercury column in a range of 0–60 mm Hg. The BP is then taken in a standard manner and the points of the systolic and diastolic pressures are recorded. The true zero-level mercury BP is determined and subtracted from the measured pressure to yield the actual BP reading.

De Gaudemaris and colleagues [12] found that the readings of the random-zero sphygmomanometer were systematically lower than those of the standard mercury sphygmomanometer. The differential parallax error and mercury column height were considered to explain the difference, but the exact reasons for the difference in readings between the two sphygmomanometers are still unclear. It is therefore recommended that these two methods not be used interchangeably in epidemiologic studies.

Infrasonic

The Infrasonic is a physiometric device that uses a filtered, low-frequency sensing transducer placed underneath an occluding cuff. The vibrations of the Korotkoff sounds are transmitted to the transducer and converted to electronic signals that are recorded on a circular disc paper. This device presents two major problems, each arising from the manufacturer's recommended use of the oversized cuff. First, if the subject's arm circumference is too small the BP level will be underestimated. Second, when compared with a mercury manometer, this device produces significantly low absolute diastolic phase IV BP readings.

Voors and colleagues [13] performed validation studies comparing the physiometric instrument with the conventional mercury sphygmomanometer. The systolic and diastolic pressure readings using the physiometric recorder were lower in younger children and higher in older children when compared to the readings of the standard mercury sphygmomanometer. Additionally, there was a large difference between the two methods in BP readings of black children. Overall, when compared with the Doppler ultrasound, infrasonic performed inferiorly [14].

Factors Affecting Blood Pressure Measurement

Several variables have been shown to alter BP levels. Bladder cuff size has already been discussed.

In addition, BP levels vary depending on the time the procedure is done. Millar-Craig and co-authors [15] found that adult BP was highest mid-morning and then fell progressively throughout the day. Prineas and colleagues [16] showed that systolic BP measurements in children were lower in the morning than in the afternoon. On the other hand, Canner and colleagues [17] found only a minuscule effect of time of day. Rose showed seasonal variation of BP levels [18]. The temperature of the examination room can also affect BP level. In their study of 9,977 children, Prineas and colleagues [16] found that with warmer temperatures diastolic BP was higher, while systolic BP was lower. The recommended examination room temperature is 68–76°F.

Other factors that may influence BP levels include: (1) place of examination [19], (2) the subject's position [20], (3) the type of sphygmomanometer used [21], (4) the position of the arm [22], and (5) whether the DBP4 or DBP5 is used to characterize diastolic BP [23, 24].

Ambulatory Blood Pressure Monitoring

BP changes continually throughout the day and night in response to changes in activity [24]. The development of automatic ambulatory BP monitoring (ABPM) enables one to measure BP throughout a 24-hour period even during routine activities. The equipment uses a standard BP cuff taped around the upper arm. The BP is recorded either by oscillometry or by auscultation, which uses a microphone. The signals from the transducer or microphone are stored on tape or a solid-state memory. Calibration of the device by simultaneous BP measurement with a standard manometer should be performed before the initiation of the 24-hour recording.

The parameters that can be programmed are the frequency of BP measurements and the rate of pressure release (or bleed step). The BPs are measured every 20–30 minutes during the day and every 30–60 minutes at night to avoid sleep disturbance. A bleed step of 8 mm Hg is as accurate as a slower rate of release and is better tolerated by pediatric patients [25].

The data are then evaluated for the mean systolic and diastolic BP over the 24-hour period. In adult patients, the upper limit of normal is

140/90 for daytime, 120/80 for nighttime, and 135/85 for the whole day. No normal values are yet available for children. Portman and Yetman [26] use the age- and gender-appropriate ninety-fifth percentile from the Task Force Study as the daytime upper limit of normal and 10% lower percentile for the upper limit at night.

Some of the primary advantages of ABPM include no alerting response, no placebo effect, multiple measurements over a 24-hour period, evaluation of long-term (diurnal) variability, measurement of BP during both usual activity and sleep, and reduction in treatment of mild hypertension [27]. It also avoids the effect of "white coat hypertension," or hypertension only in the presence of health care workers, which is common in both adults and children. Hornsby and colleagues [28] found that 44% of pediatric patients (ages 5–15) found to be hypertensive using standard office BP devices were reclassified as normotensive when assessed with ABPM.

Several data have shown that ABPM provides the best correlation between BP and left ventricular hypertrophy (LVH) [29–31]. White and colleagues [32] found that in adult patients, the average daily BP obtained by the ABPM correlated with the left ventricular mass index but did not correlate with office BP. Several investigations, however, have found different results when correlating BP with LVH. Verdecchia and colleagues [31] found that LVH correlated better with BP during nighttime. On the other hand, Devereaux [33] found a closer correlation between BP and LVH during routine working hours.

ABPM has been shown to be well tolerated and easily accomplished in the pediatric population [25]. However, normal values must be established and the technique must be standardized for children. Also, because the device detects only the phase V, and not the phase IV, Korotkoff sound, the diastolic BP reading will be lower in children less than 13 years of age.

Definition and Classification of Hypertension

The Report of the Second Task Force on Blood Pressure Control in Children provided data on the normal distribution of BP from birth to maturity [5]. In addition, the report established a set of standards for diagnosing hypertension in a young individual and developed age- and sex-specific curves (Figure 2.3). The most powerful determinant of normal BP change is maturation, not chronologic age [34]. In addition, BP does not correlate with age when height and body mass index are considered [35]. Rosner and colleagues provided normative BP data using height as the index of maturation (Tables 2.2 and 2.3) [36]. Using these new standards, more short children and fewer tall children are classified as hypertensive.

The Task Force also set guidelines for the definition of hypertension [5]. *Normal BP* is defined as systolic and diastolic levels less than the ninetieth percentile for age and sex; *high normal BP* is defined as average

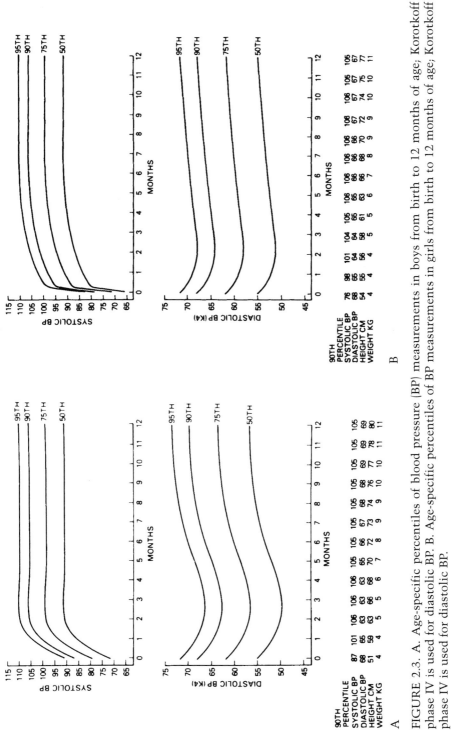

FIGURE 2.3. A. Age-specific percentiles of blood pressure (BP) measurements in boys from birth to 12 months of age; Korotkoff phase IV is used for diastolic BP. B. Age-specific percentiles of BP measurements in girls from birth to 12 months of age; Korotkoff phase IV is used for diastolic BP.

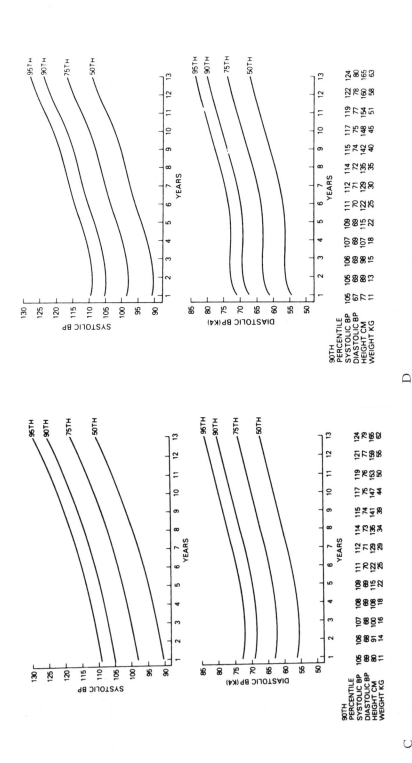

FIGURE 2.3 *(continued)* C. Age-specific percentiles of BP measurements in boys from 1 to 13 years of age; Korotkoff phase IV is used for diastolic BP. D. Age-specific percentiles of BP measurements in girls from 1 to 13 years of age; Korotkoff phase IV is used for diastolic BP.

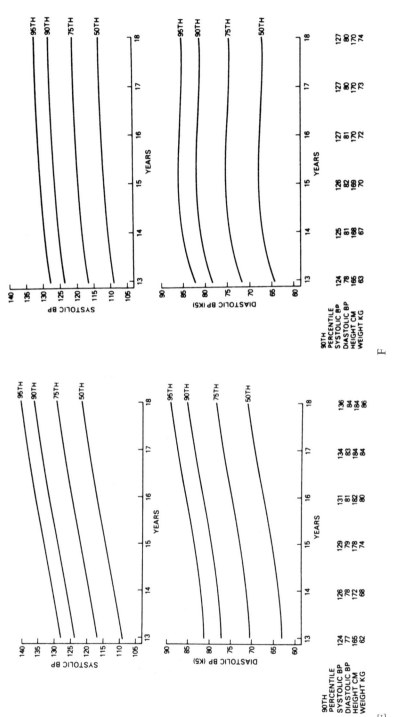

FIGURE 2.3 *(continued)* E. Age-specific percentiles of BP measurements in boys from 13 to 18 years of age; Korotkoff phase V is used for diastolic BP. F. Age-specific percentiles of BP measurements in girls from 13 to 18 years of age; Korotkoff phase V is used for diastolic BP. (Reproduced with permission from Report of the Second Task Force on Blood Pressure Control in Children—1987. Pediatrics 1987;79:1.)

TABLE 2.2
Blood Pressure Levels for the Ninetieth and Ninety-Fifth Percentiles of Blood Pressure for Boys 1–17 Years of Age (Stratified by Percentiles of Height)

Age	Percentile	Systolic BP (mm Hg) by Percentile of Height							Diastolic BP (mm Hg) by Percentile of Height						
		5%	10%	25%	50%	75%	90%	95%	5%	10%	25%	50%	75%	90%	95%
1	90th	94	95	97	99	101	102	103	49	49	50	51	52	53	54
	95th	98	99	101	103	105	106	107	54	54	55	56	57	58	58
2	90th	98	99	101	103	104	106	107	54	54	55	56	57	58	58
	95th	102	103	105	107	108	110	110	58	59	60	61	62	63	63
3	90th	101	102	103	105	107	109	109	59	59	60	61	62	63	63
	95th	105	106	107	109	111	112	113	63	63	64	65	66	67	68
4	90th	103	104	105	107	109	110	111	63	63	64	65	66	67	67
	95th	107	108	109	111	113	114	115	67	68	68	69	70	71	72
5	90th	104	105	107	109	111	112	113	66	67	68	69	70	71	71
	95th	108	109	111	113	114	116	117	71	71	72	73	74	75	76
6	90th	105	106	108	110	112	113	114	70	70	71	72	73	74	74
	95th	109	110	112	114	116	117	118	74	75	75	76	77	78	79
7	90th	106	107	109	111	113	114	115	72	73	73	74	75	76	77
	95th	110	111	113	115	117	118	119	77	77	78	79	80	81	81
8	90th	108	109	110	112	114	116	116	74	75	75	76	77	78	79
	95th	112	113	114	116	118	119	120	79	79	80	81	82	83	83

				Systolic								Diastolic				
9	90th	109	110	112	114	116	117	118	76	76	77	78	79	80	80
	95th	113	114	116	118	119	121	122	80	81	81	82	83	84	85
10	90th	111	112	113	115	117	119	119	77	77	78	79	80	81	81
	95th	115	116	117	119	121	123	123	81	82	83	83	84	85	86
11	90th	113	114	115	117	119	121	121	77	78	79	80	81	81	81
	95th	117	118	119	121	123	125	125	82	82	83	84	85	86	86
12	90th	115	116	118	120	121	123	124	78	78	79	80	81	82	82
	95th	119	120	122	124	125	127	128	83	83	84	85	86	87	87
13	90th	118	119	120	122	124	125	126	78	79	80	81	81	82	83
	95th	121	122	124	126	128	129	130	83	83	84	85	86	87	88
14	90th	120	121	123	125	127	128	129	79	79	80	81	82	83	83
	95th	124	125	127	129	131	132	133	83	84	85	86	87	87	88
15	90th	123	124	126	128	130	131	132	80	80	81	82	83	84	84
	95th	127	128	130	132	133	135	136	84	85	86	86	87	88	89
16	90th	126	127	129	131	132	134	134	81	82	82	83	84	85	86
	95th	130	131	133	134	136	138	138	86	86	86	88	89	90	90
17	90th	128	129	131	133	135	136	137	83	84	85	86	87	87	88
	95th	132	133	135	137	139	140	141	88	88	89	90	91	92	93

Source: Reproduced with permission from B Rosner, RJ Prineas, JM Loggie, SR Daniels. Blood pressure nomogram for children and adolescents, by height, sex, and age, in the United States. J Pediatr 1993;123:871.

TABLE 2.3
Blood Pressure Levels for the Ninetieth and Ninety-Fifth Percentiles of Blood Pressure for Girls 1–17 Years of Age (Stratified by Percentiles of Height)

Age (yr)	Percentile	Systolic BP (mm HG) by percentile of height							Diastolic BP (mm HG) by percentile of height						
		5%	10%	25%	50%	75%	90%	95%	5%	10%	25%	50%	75%	90%	95%
1	90th	98	98	99	101	102	103	104	52	52	53	53	54	55	55
	95th	101	102	103	104	106	107	108	56	56	57	58	58	59	60
2	90th	99	99	101	102	103	104	105	57	57	58	58	59	60	60
	95th	103	103	104	106	107	108	109	61	61	62	62	63	64	64
3	90th	100	101	102	103	104	105	106	61	61	61	62	63	64	64
	95th	104	104	106	107	108	109	110	65	65	66	66	67	68	68
4	90th	101	102	103	104	106	107	108	64	64	65	65	66	67	67
	95th	105	106	107	108	109	111	111	68	68	69	69	70	71	71
5	90th	103	103	105	106	107	108	109	66	67	67	68	69	69	70
	95th	107	107	108	110	111	112	113	71	71	71	72	73	74	74
6	90th	104	105	106	107	109	110	111	69	69	69	70	71	72	72
	95th	108	109	110	111	113	114	114	73	73	74	74	75	76	76
7	90th	106	107	108	109	110	112	112	71	71	71	72	73	74	74
	95th	110	111	112	113	114	115	116	75	75	75	76	77	78	78

Age				Systolic							Diastolic				
8	90th	108	109	110	111	112	114	114	72	72	73	74	74	75	76
	95th	112	113	114	115	116	117	118	76	77	77	78	79	79	80
9	90th	110	111	112	113	114	116	116	74	74	74	75	76	77	77
	95th	114	115	116	117	118	119	120	78	78	78	79	80	81	81
10	90th	112	113	114	115	116	118	118	75	75	76	77	77	78	78
	95th	116	117	118	119	120	122	122	79	79	80	81	81	82	83
11	90th	114	115	116	117	119	120	120	76	77	77	78	79	79	80
	95th	118	119	120	121	122	124	124	81	81	81	82	83	83	84
12	90th	116	117	118	119	121	122	123	78	78	78	79	80	81	81
	95th	120	121	122	123	125	126	126	82	82	82	83	84	85	85
13	90th	118	119	120	121	123	124	124	79	79	79	80	81	82	82
	95th	122	123	124	125	126	128	128	83	83	84	84	85	86	86
14	90th	120	121	122	123	124	125	126	80	80	80	81	82	83	83
	95th	124	125	126	127	128	129	130	84	84	85	85	86	87	87
15	90th	121	122	123	124	126	127	128	80	80	81	82	83	83	84
	95th	125	126	127	128	130	131	131	85	85	85	86	87	88	88
16	90th	122	123	124	125	127	128	129	81	81	82	82	83	84	84
	95th	126	127	128	129	130	132	132	85	85	86	87	87	88	88
17	90th	123	123	124	126	127	128	129	81	81	82	83	83	84	85
	95th	127	127	128	130	131	132	133	85	86	86	87	88	88	89

Source: Reproduced with permission from B Rosner, RJ Prineas, JM Loggie, SR Daniels. Blood pressure nomogram for children and adolescents, by height, sex, and age, in the United States. J Pediatr 1993;123:871.

systolic and/or diastolic BP between the ninetieth and ninety-fifth percentiles for age and sex; and *hypertension* is defined as average systolic and diastolic BP equal or greater than the ninety-fifth percentile for age and sex with measurements taken on at least three occasions. Using a bedside pearl (Alan Gruskin Criteria), hypertension (>ninety-fifth percentile) in pediatrics can be defined as the point at which:

The systolic BP > 100 + [3.0 × patient's age in years]

or

The diastolic BP > 70 + [1.5 × patient's age in years]

or

The BP > 140/90 for adolescents 14 years or older

Classification of hypertension in adults—mild, moderate, or severe—is generally based on the diastolic BP level. Mild hypertension occurs when the diastolic BP is 90–100 mm Hg, moderate occurs at 100–110 mm Hg, and severe occurs at greater than 110 mm Hg. For children, the classification based on age has been provided by the Task Force (Table 2.4). Of note, the differential increase from significant hypertension to severe hypertension is not that great.

A bedside pearl (Alan Gruskin Criteria) for classification of hypertension in pediatrics is:

Mild hypertension: Blood pressure is 1–15% above the ninety-fifth percentile for age/sex

Moderate hypertension: Blood pressure is 16–30% above the ninety-fifth percentile for age/sex

Severe hypertension: Blood pressure is 31–50% above the ninety-fifth percentile for age/sex

Emergency: Blood pressure is >50% above the ninety-fifth percentile for age/sex

The Task Force also produced guidelines for the systemic identification of children with elevated BP measurements [5]. With the exception of severe hypertension with manifestations of end-organ damage, identification of children with elevated BPs requires multiple determinations on several visits. If the BP value is above the ninety-fifth percentile for the child's age and sex, the child is scheduled for repeat BP measurements over several visits (every 1–2 weeks). If the average BP reading is below the ninetieth percentile, the child resumes continuing health care. For average BP measurements at the ninety-fifth percentile or higher, the patient should be diagnostically evaluated and consideration should be given to therapy. However, if the child is obese (see Chapter 7), a trial of weight control may be tried before proceeding to a referral, diagnostic evaluation, and other therapies.

TABLE 2.4
Classification of Hypertension by Age Group

Age Group	Significant Hypertension (mm Hg)	Severe Hypertension (mm Hg)
Newborn		
7 days	Systolic BP ≥96	Systolic BP≥106
8–30 days	Systolic BP ≥104	Systolic BP≥110
Infant (<2 yrs)	Systolic BP ≥112	Systolic BP ≥118
	Diastolic BP ≥74	Diastolic BP ≥82
Children (3–5 yrs)	Systolic BP ≥116	Systolic BP ≥124
	Diastolic BP ≥76	Diastolic BP ≥84
Children (6–9 yrs)	Systolic BP ≥122	Systolic BP ≥130
	Diastolic BP ≥78	Diastolic BP ≥86
Children (10–12 yrs)	Systolic BP ≥126	Systolic BP ≥134
	Diastolic BP ≥82	Diastolic BP ≥90
Adolescents (13–15 yrs)	Systolic BP ≥136	Systolic BP ≥144
	Diastolic BP ≥86	Diastolic BP ≥92
Adolescents (16–18 yrs)	Systolic BP ≥142	Systolic BP ≥150
	Diastolic BP ≥92	Diastolic BP ≥98

Source: Reproduced with permission from Report of the Second Task Force on Blood Pressure Control in Children—1987. Pediatrics 1987;79:1.

The height and weight for the ninetieth percentile for age (displayed at the bottom of each age/BP graph) is consulted if the average BP reading is between the ninetieth and ninety-fifth percentile for age. The child returns to continuing health care if he or she is tall and not obese or the weight is above the ninetieth percentile because of an increase in lean body mass. Weight control is recommended with BP monitoring for a BP reading that is above the ninetieth percentile because of obesity. For BP readings between the ninetieth and ninety-fifth percentile that cannot be accounted for by either excess weight or height for age, the child should remain under surveillance and BP should be monitored at least every 6 months.

It is also recommended by the Task Force [5] that the child's BP be recorded and plotted on the BP/age percentile charts. This helps to determine at a glance which curve the child's BP is following and will provide guidance as to how closely the BP should be monitored.

Prevalence of Hypertension

Prevalence is defined as the proportion of population who have a disease at one point in time. Hypertension with no known cause is classified as

TABLE 2.5
Conditions Suggesting Increased Hypertension Risk for Infants

---

Abdominal bruit
Abdominal mass(es) (e.g., Wilms' tumor, neuroblastoma)
Certain acute clinical situations (e.g., burns, hemolytic uremic syndrome)
Coarctation of the aorta
Congenital adrenal hyperplasia
Neurofibromatosis
Failure to grow
Indwelling umbilical catheter
Administration of glucocorticoids and/or adrenocorticotropic hormone
Orbital tumor
Suspected renal disease (hematuria, proteinuria)
Turner syndrome
Unexplained heart failure
Unexplained seizures

---

essential or *primary*, while *secondary hypertension* is the term used to described an abnormally elevated BP caused by an illness, diseased organ, or anatomic anomaly.

The estimated prevalence of essential hypertension in the adult population is about 15–20%. In infants and preschool children, the prevalence is still not known, and identifiable hypertension is usually due to an underlying cause. The most common cause of hypertension for neonates is renovascular disease; for older children, it is renal disease. Several conditions may suggest an increased risk of hypertension (Table 2.5) [37].

The data on the prevalence of essential hypertension in older children and adolescents are variable. They have been reported as both 1–2% [38] and 5% [39]. In the study by Sinaiko and colleagues [40] on 14,686 school children ages 10–15, approximately 5% had significant systolic and diastolic hypertension after initial screening. However, after the rescreening examination, the percentage of students with significant hypertension was reduced to about 1%. This report shows the importance of repeated BP measurements to make an accurate diagnosis of hypertension.

There are few data on prevalence rates for secondary hypertension in older children and adolescents. Some of the causes of secondary hypertension include renal parenchymal disease, renovascular disease, cardiovascular disease, and the endocrinopathies. For the majority of severe symptomatic hypertension, an underlying organic disease is usually responsible [41]. For asymptomatic patients, Loggie [42] recommended a workup if the child is less than 10 years of age because of the high probability of an underlying cause.

TABLE 2.6
Possible Ideal Cuff Size

Midpoint Upper Arm Circumference (cm)	Bladder Width (cm) 33–43% of Arm Circumference	Bladdder Width (cm) >90% of Arm Circumference
14–15	6	16
19–24	8	22
25–30	10	27
31–39	13	35
40–52	17	47

Source: Modified from RJ Prineas, ZM Elkwiry. Epidemiology and Measurement of High Blood Pressure in Children and Adolescents. In JMH Loggie (ed), Pediatric and Adolescent Hypertension. Boston: Blackwell, 1992. Reprinted by permission of Blackwell Scientific Publications, Inc.

Epidemiology of Hypertension

In adults, hypertension has been shown to be a risk factor for atherosclerotic vascular disease, stroke, and renal disease. In children, it may be a sign of essential hypertension or a manifestation of a correctable underlying organ dysfunction. It is important to understand the circumstances and factors involved in high BP readings.

Blood Pressure Measurement

Bladder Cuff Size

It has always been emphasized that the correct bladder and cuff size based on the subject's extremities should be used to avoid erroneous readings. This is also true for neonates and infants. The extremities of children, including neonates and infants, vary at different ages and grow at different rates. A correct bladder and cuff size, based on the subject's extremities, should be used to avoid erroneous readings. The Minneapolis Children's Blood Pressure Study recommended the use of a cuff bladder width that is greater than 120% of the diameter of the extremity [16]. Prineas and Elkwiry [43] made a different proposal on the ideal bladder width for older children and adolescents as shown in Table 2.6. They based the bladder width on the arm circumference and not on the arm length. The calculated width is 33–43% of the arm circumference. There are fewer data on the standard specification for bladder length. In a study of 50 adults, Burch and Shewey [44] suggested that the bladder need only encircle one-half the circumference of the arm. On the other hand, Voors [45], in a study of 443 grade school children, found that deficient bladder length was associated with elevated BP readings. The Minnesota Children's Blood Pressure Study recommended that the bladder cuff encircle at least 90% of the arm's circumference [16].

Measuring Device

Doppler ultrasound is useful for infant BP measurement. The readings have been shown to closely resemble direct intra-arterial measurements [10, 46]. This device has been recommended for BP studies of children less than 2 years of age.

For older children and adolescents, the standard mercury sphygmomanometer has been used for epidemiologic studies. The random-zero sphygmomanometer has also been recommended to remove the observer bias for digit preference of BP reading. However, it should not be used interchangeably with the standard mercury sphygmomanometer when undergoing epidemiologic studies.

Age

BP in infants increases with age. During the first 5 days after birth, it has been shown to rise considerably from 59 to 90 mm Hg systolic BP and from 43 to 55 mm Hg diastolic BP [47]. The mean systolic BP continues to increase at 6 weeks of age but shows little further change between 6 months and 1 year [48, 49]. BP levels tend to reach a plateau at 6–15 months, when BP is about 1–2 mm Hg higher than BP at 6 months of age. Compared to the readings at 1 year of age, at 2 years of age the systolic BP is about 4 mm Hg higher and the diastolic BP is about 2 mm Hg higher [50]. It was noted that the BP was about 6 mm Hg higher for awake babies than those who were sleeping [48].

For older children and adolescents, systolic BP rises at a rate of about 1–2 mm Hg per year from the age of 5, while diastolic BP increases at a degree of 0.5–1.0 mm Hg per year [43]. The 1987 Report of the Second Task Force on Blood Pressure in Children provides comprehensive data on the BP distribution by age of infants, older children, and adolescents [5].

Kahn and colleagues [51] have shown that with the use of vertex-corrected mean arterial pressure (VMAP), there is no linear association between BP and age. They did, however, demonstrate a linear correlation between BP and ponderousness. The VMAP was based on the principle that the active perfusion of the brain requires the BP at the heart level to exceed the hydrostatic pressure defined by the distance between the heart and the head (Figure 2.4). This is best illustrated by the giraffe, which has an elongated neck that contributes to a very long hydrostatic column against which the heart must pump to perfuse the brain. The standing giraffe requires a BP range from 260/158 to 340/303 mm Hg [52]. In the study by Kahn and colleagues [51], the cuff-to-vertex (top of subject's head) length is recorded and the height is converted to its equivalent in mm Hg. The value is then subtracted from the BP value observed at the cuff. The mean VMAP for 6- to 13-year-old boys was 49.4 mm Hg. For 14- to 17-year-old boys, it was 46.0 mm Hg. For 6- to 17-year-old girls, the mean VMAP was 50.2 mm Hg [51].

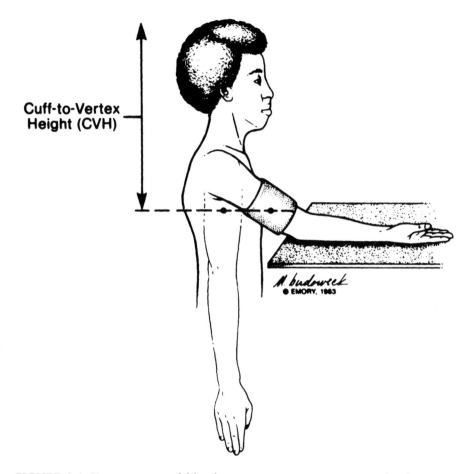

**Cuff-to-Vertex
Height (CVH)**

FIGURE 2.4. Vertex-corrected blood pressure measurements use the distance in centimeters from the midpoint of the upper arm to the top of the head (CVH) to dampen blood pressure variability due to age and height. (Vertex-corrected blood pressure = measured blood pressure – 0.779 [CVH]). (Reproduced with permission from HS Kahn, RP Bain. Vertex-corrected blood pressure in black girls. Hypertension 1987;9:390.)

Sex

In the first two years of age, several studies have shown no significant difference in BP between males and females [47, 49, 53–55]. However, in the studies by Hennekens and colleagues [56] and Levine and colleagues [57], boys are shown to have slightly higher BP than girls. De Swiet and colleagues [48] also found a slightly higher BP in boys who were heavier; however, the difference was eliminated after the BP readings were adjusted for weight.

The 1987 Report of the Second Task Force on Blood Pressure Control in Children [5] provided the distribution of systolic and diastolic BP for boys and girls through 18 years of age. It should be noted that for the diastolic BP for children less than 13 years of age, the phase IV Korotkoff sound was used, and for 13- to 18-year-old adolescents, the phase V Korotkoff sound was used. There are only minimal differences of BP levels between boys and girls until 13 years of age. Thereafter, at ages 13–18 years, it is noted that the BP levels for boys increase more steeply than for girls.

Race

The prevalence of hypertension in black adults in the United States is about 25%. The influence of race on hypertension in blacks and whites during the first 2 years of life is not known [49].

The Bogalusa Heart Study found little difference in BP levels between Hispanic, white, and black children [58]. Several other studies also did not find any differences in BPs between black and white children [59, 60]. Baron and colleagues [61] found that black boys 13–18 years old did not show significant differences in BP when compared with whites and Mexican-Americans, but girls in the same age group have slightly higher systolic BP levels.

A meta-analysis of 35 studies on the racial differences of BP in children was conducted by Alpert and Fox [62]. Six of the 35 studies showed no racial differences. Table 2.7 summarizes the remaining 29 studies in which racial differences were found. Diastolic BP in black boys was higher than those of whites and Asians. The analysis also showed a significantly higher BP, both systolic and diastolic, in black girls.

Several factors have been associated with the variations in BP levels, though the exact mechanism is not known. These include differences in diet, plasma-renin levels, sodium excretion, and socio-economic factors. Studies have also shown differences in salt sensitivity between blacks and whites. In adults, both hypertensive and normotensive blacks have a higher prevalence of BP response to sodium loading than whites [63]. Dimsdale and co-authors [64] showed that blacks have a higher pressor sensitivity to an increased salt diet when compared to whites.

Familial Aggregation

Familial aggregation, which has been demonstrated in infants, points to the importance of genetic influences on the BP levels in children. It may be due to gene effects, shared environments, or an interaction of these two factors. The correlation for the genetic variance of BP was shown to be higher in monozygotic than dizygotic twins [65, 66]. Another study on twins by Levine and co-authors [54] found a statistically significant genetic variance for systolic BP at 6 months of age. The data suggested that genetic effects on BP within a family may be detected early in life.

TABLE 2.7
Meta-Analysis of Race, Age, and Sex Subgroups

Sex	Age (yrs)	Measure	Racial Comparison	p value
Males	0–12	DBP	B>C	$p <0.034$
		SBP	H>C	$p <0.061$
		DBP	B>A	$p <0.055$
		DBP	A>H	$p <0.04$
Females	0–12	SBP	B>A	$p <0.071$
	13–18	SBP	B>C	$p <0.099$
		SBP	B>H	$p <0.048$
	19–25	DBP	B>C	$p <0.086$

B = black; C = caucasian; H = hispanic; A = Asian; SBP = systolic blood pressure; DBP= diastolic blood pressure.
Source: Modified from BS Albert, ME Fox. Racial aspects of blood pressure in children and adolescents. Pediatr Clin North Am 1993;40:16.

Zinner and others [53] likewise found that infant BP correlated with maternal BP shortly after birth, while father–infant correlations were significant only at 1 month of age. The data also showed significant correlation between siblings at 6 months of age. Another study by Hennekens and colleagues [56] involved the evaluation of BP in 93 siblings from 43 black families with newborns. Their data showed a sib-sib intraclass correlation of 0.26 for systolic and 0.16 for diastolic pressure. A greater variance of BP was demonstrated between families than among members of the same family [56].

There seem to be a variation of reports on the correlation between parent–sibling BPs. Munger and co-authors [67] reported higher correlations of BP between mothers and children. In Mexican-American families, Paterson and colleagues [68] found significant correlations between fathers' and childrens' BPs.

Shared environment has also been shown to play a role in the familial aggregation of BP. The Montreal Adoption Study enrolled 1,176 parents, 756 adopted children, and 445 children and their natural parents to study the influence of genes and household environment. The survey showed that shared genes accounted for 58% of the variance of diastolic BP, while 42% of the variance was shown to be caused by environment shared across the generations. Perruse and others [69] have also shown that familial environment accounts for a substantial proportion of variability in BP.

There are substantial data to support a familial component to BP and hypertension. Several studies have suggested the possibility of a gene that could dictate the BP level of an individual. Controversy still remains as to whether there is a major gene modified by environmental factors. Miyao and Furusho [70] examined the possible mode of inheritance of hypertension between hypertensive and normotensive parents in the Japanese offspring of different partners. Depending on the geographic location of the study, if one parent was hypertensive, the incidence of hypertension in children ranged from 15.9% to 56.8%, and for two hypertensive parents it ranged from 44.0% to 73.3%. These results do not spell out the risk of hypertension for an individual child. They concluded that essential hypertension is a polygenic disease governed by polygenic systems, and that inheritance and environment are of equal importance as factors for its appearance.

The length of stay in an environment could play a part in the familial aggregation of BP. Data on other factors on the environment such as shared family stress, shared caloric intake, or shared salt intake are still inadequate. Manipulation of these factors may give the caregiver the chance to alter the course of hypertension in a child with a strong family history and even prevent its future occurrence.

Blood Pressure Tracking

BP has been shown to increase from infancy to adolescence. The possibility that adult hypertension starts during childhood has been suggested by several studies. *BP tracking* has been defined as maintenance of BP in relation to peers in order to predict BP later in life.

How the infant BP will predict future hypertension is still unknown. Zinner and associates [53] did not find BPs of infants less than 6 months of age to be predictive of later pressures, but showed significant correlations for both systolic and diastolic BPs at 6 and 12 months of age. Schachter and colleagues [49] followed up the BP readings of 3-day-old babies at 6, 15, and 24 months. Significant tracking correlations for systolic BP were found with correlations ranging from 0.23 to 0.32.

The Bogalusa Heart Study [71] measured the BP of 440 children from birth to 7 years of age. The data demonstrated that significant prediction of BP at 7 years of age could occur at 6 months of age for systolic BP ($r = 0.24$ for correlation with year 1). For diastolic BP, consistent prediction did not occur until 1 year of age ($r = 0.14$ for correlation with year 2). In the study involving children 5–14 years of age observed over 3 years [73], the year 1 to year 4 correlations ranged from 0.52–0.63 for systolic BP and from 0.23–0.45 for diastolic phase IV BP.

The Muscatine Study [72], which sampled school-age children, showed a 6-year correlation for systolic BP of 0.30 and a correlation of 0.18 for diastolic BP. Higgins and others [74] demonstrated that initial BP for children 6–19 years old is one of the predictors of high systolic BP after re-examination at an average interval of 13 years. The data also showed that improvement of prediction in boys increased with age. The observation of better projection in boys has also been noted by Woynarowska and colleagues [75]. The data showed significant associations between BP levels at 9 years of age and at 30 years of age for systolic BP in male subjects. The association with diastolic BP was not significant.

The tracking data on BP have shown the possibility of predicting BP levels as early as infancy. However, the value of BP at infancy for predicting future hypertension is still unknown. Gillman and colleagues [76] re-examined, 8–12 years later, the BPs in children initially seen at 8–15 years of age. Their data showed that the resulting sensitivities and predictive values of childhood BP as a screening test for adult BP are only of modest magnitude. Their data also questioned the usefulness of routine BP measurement to identify children at high risk for development of essential hypertension.

References

1. RM Berne, M Levy (eds). Physiology (3rd ed). St Louis: Mosby-Year Book, 1993.
2. Steinfeld L, Alexander H, Cohen ML. Updating sphygmomanometry. Am J Cardiol 1974;33:107.
3. Kirkendall WM, Feinleib M, Freis ED, Mark AL. Recommendations for human blood pressure determinations by sphygmomanometers (AHA Committee Report). Circulation 1980;62:1149.
4. Prineas RJ, Jacobs D. Quality of Korotkoff sounds: bell vs diaphragm, cubital fossa vs brachial artery. Prev Med 1983;12:715.
5. Report of the Second Task Force on Blood Pressure Control in Children—1987. Pediatrics 1987;79:1.
6. Moss AJ, Adams FH. Problems of Blood Pressure in Childhood. Springfield, IL: Charles C. Thomas, 1962.
7. Moss AJ, Liebling W, Austin WO, Adams FH. An evaluation of the flush method for determining blood pressures in infants. Pediatrics 1957;20:53.
8. Stegall HF, Kardon MB, Kemmerer WT. Indirect measurement of arterial blood pressure by Doppler ultrasonic sphygmomanometry. J Appl Physiol 1968;25:793.
9. Gordon LS, Johnson PE, Penido JRF, et al. Systolic and diastolic measurements by transcutaneous Doppler ultrasound in premature infants in critical care nurseries and at closed heart surgery. Anesth Analg 1974;53:914.
10. Elseed AM, Shinebourne EA, Joseph MC. Assessment of techniques for measurement of blood pressure in infants and children. Arch Dis Child 1973;48:932.
11. Colan SD, Fuji A, Borow KM, et al. Noninvasive determination of systolic, diastolic, and end-systolic blood pressure in neonates, infants and young children: comparison with central aortic pressure measurements. Am J Cardiol 1983;52:867.

12. De Gaudemaris R, Folsom AR, Prineas RJ, Luepker RV. The random-zero versus the standard mercury sphygmomanometer: a systematic blood pressure difference. Am J Epidemiol 1985;121:282.

13. Voors AW, Foster TH, Frerichs RR, et al. The Bogalusa Heart Study—studies of blood pressure in children, ages 5–14 years, in a total biracial community. Circulation 1976;54:319.

14. Reder RF, Dimich I, Cohen ML, Steinfeld L. Evaluating indirect blood pressure measurement techniques: a comparison of three systems in infants and children. Pediatrics 1978;62:326.

15. Millar-Craig MW, Bishop CN, Raferty EB. Circadian variation of blood pressure. Lancet 1978;1:795.

16. Prineas RJ, Gillum RF, Horibe H, Hannan PJ. The Minneapolis Children's Blood Pressure Study—Part 1: Standards of measurement for children's blood pressure. Hypertension 1980;2:18.

17. Canner PL, Borhani NO, Oberman A, et al. The hypertension prevention trial: assessment of the quality of blood pressure measurements. Am J Epidemiol 1991;134:379.

18. Rose G. Seasonal variation in blood pressure in man [letter]. Nature 1961;189:235.

19. Gillum RF, Etemadi N, Boen JR, et al. Home versus clinic blood pressure measurements. J Natl Med Assoc 1982;74:545.

20. Gauer OH, Thron HL. Postural Changes in Circulation. In WF Hamilton (ed), Circulation (vol 3). Washington: American Physiological Society, 1965;2409.

21. Mitchell PL, Parlin RW, Blackburn H. Effect of vertical displacement of the arm on indirect blood pressure measurement. N Engl J Med 1964;271:72.

22. Sinaiko AR, Gomez-Marin O, Prineas R. Diastolic fourth and fifth phase blood pressure in 10–15 year old children: The Children and Adolescent Blood Pressure Program. Am J Epidemiol 1990;132:647.

23. Folsom AR, Prineas RJ, Jacobs DR, et al. Measured differences between fourth and fifth phase diastolic blood pressure in 4,885 adults: implications for blood pressure surveys. Int J Epidemiol 1984;13:436.

24. James GD, Pickering TG. The influence of behavioral factors on daily variation of blood pressure. Am J Hypertens 1993;6:170.

25. Portman RJ, Yetman RJ, West MS. Efficacy of 24-hour ABPM in children. J Pediatr 1991;118:842.

26. Portman RJ, Yetman RJ. Clinical uses of ABPM. Pediatr Nephrol 1994;8:367.

27. Meyer-Sabellek W, Schulte KL, Gotzen R. Non-invasive ABPM: technical possibilities and problems. J Hypertens 1990;8:3.

28. Hornsby JL, Mongan PF, Taylor AT, Treiber FA. "White coat" hypertension in children. J Fam Pract 1991;33:617.

29. White WB, Dey HM, Schulman P. Assessment of the daily blood pressure load as a determinant of cardiac function in patients with mild-to-moderate hypertension. Am Heart J 1989;118:782.

30. Perloff D, Sokolow M, Cowan RM, Juster RP. Prognostic value of ambulatory blood pressure measurements: further analysis. J Hypertens 1989;7:3.

31. Verdecchia P, Schillaci G, Guerrieri M, et al. Circadian blood pressure changes and left ventricular hypertrophy in essential hypertension. Circulation 1990;81:528.

32. White WB, Schulman P, McCabe EJ, Dey HM. Average daily blood pressure, not office blood pressure, determines cardiac function in patients with hypertension. JAMA 1989;261:873.

33. Devereaux RB, Pickering TG, Harshfield GA, et al. Left ventricular hypertrophy in patients with hypertension: importance of blood pressure response to regularly recurring stress. Circulation 1983;68:470.

34. Gillum RF, Prineas RJ, Horibe H. Maturation vs age: assessing blood pressure by height. J Natl Med Assoc 1982;74:43.

35. Voors AW, Weber LS, Frerichs RR, Berenson GS. Body height and body mass as determinants of basal blood pressure in children—the Bogalusa Heart Study. Am J Epidemiol 1977;106:101.

36. Rosner B, Prineas RJ, Loggie JM, Daniels SR. Blood pressure nomogram for children and adolescents, by height, sex, and age, in the United States. J Pediatr 1993;123:871.

37. McCrory WW. Definition, Prevalence and Distribution of Causes of Hypertension. In JMH Loggie (ed), Pediatric and Adolescent Hypertension. Boston: Blackwell, 1992.

38. Fixler DE, Laird WP, Fitzgerald V, Stead S, Adams R. Hypertension screening in schools: Results of the Dallas study. Pediatrics 1979;63:32.

39. Loggie JM. Evaluation and management of childhood hypertension. Surg Clin North Am 1985;65:1623.

40. Sinaiko AR, Gomez-Marin O, Prineas RJ. Prevalence of "significant" hypertension in junior high school-aged children: The Children and Adolescent Blood Pressure Program. J Pediatr 1989;114:664.

41. Londe S. Causes of hypertension in the young. Pediatr Clin North Am 1978;25:55.

42. Loggie JMH. Hypertension in children and adolescents. Hosp Pract (Off Ed) 1975;132:81.

43. Prineas RJ, Elkwiry ZM. Epidemiology and Measurement of High Blood Pressure in Children and Adolescents. In JMH Loggie (ed), Pediatric and Adolescent Hypertension. Boston: Blackwell, 1992.

44. Burch GE, Shewey L. Sphygmomanometric cuff size and blood pressure recordings. JAMA 1973;225:1215.

45. Voors AW. Cuff bladder size in a blood pressure survey of children. Am J Epidemiol 1975;101:489.

46. Hernandez A, Goldring D, Hartmann AF, et al. Measurement of blood pressure in infants and children by Doppler ultrasonic technique. Pediatrics 1971;48:788.

47. Uhari M. Changes in blood pressure during the first year of life. Acta Paediatr 1980;69:613.

48. De Swiet M, Fayers P, Shinebourne EA. Systolic blood pressure in a population of infants in the first year of life: the Brompton study. Pediatrics 1980;65:1028.

49. Schachter J, Kuller LH, Perfetti C. Blood pressure during the first two years of life. Am J Epidemiol 1982;116:29.
50. McGarvey ST, Zinner SH. Epidemiology of Blood Pressure in the First Two Years of Life. In JMH Loggie (ed), Pediatric and Adolescent Hypertension. Boston: Blackwell, 1992.
51. Kahn HS, Bain RP, Pullen-Smith B. Interpretation of children's blood pressure using physiologic height correction. J Chron Dis 1986;39:521.
52. Goetz RH, Warren JV, Gauer OH, et al. Circulation of the giraffe. Circ Res 1960;8:1049.
53. Zinner SH, Rosner B, Oh W, Kass EH. Significance of blood pressure in infancy. Familial aggregation and predictive effect on late blood pressure. Hypertension 1985;7:411.
54. Levine RS, Hennekens CH, Duncan RC, et al. Blood pressure in infant twins: birth to 6 months of age. Hypertension 1980;2:29.
55. Zinner SH, Lee YH, Rosner B, et al. Factors affecting blood pressures in newborn infants. Hypertension 1980;2:99.
56. Hennekens CH, Jesse MJ, Klein BE, et al. Aggregation of blood pressure in infants and their siblings. Am J Epidemiol 1976;103:457.
57. Levine RS, Hennekens CH, Perry A, et al. Genetic variance of blood pressure levels in infant twins. Am J Epidemiol 1982;116:759.
58. Webber LS, Harsha DW, Philipps GT, et al. Cardiovascular risk factors in Hispanic, white, and black children: the Brooks County and Bogalusa Heart studies. Am J Epidemiol 1991;133:704.
59. Schachter J, Kuller LH, Perfetti C. Blood pressure during the first five years of life: relation to ethnic group (black or white) and to parental hypertension. Am J Epidemiol 1984;119: 541.
60. Voors AW, Webber LS, Berenson GS. Blood pressure of children, ages 2½–5½ years, in a total biracial community—the Bogalusa Heart Study. Am J Epidemiol 1978;107:403.
61. Baron AE, Freyer B, Fixler DE. Longitudinal blood pressures in blacks, whites, and Mexican-Americans during childhood, adolescence, and early adulthood. Am J Epidemiol 1986;123:809.
62. Alpert BS, Fox ME. Racial aspects of blood pressure in children and adolescents. Pediatr Clin North Am 1993;40:13.
63. Sowers JR, Zemel MB, Zemel P, et al. Salt sensitivity in blacks. Salt intake and natriuretic substances. Hypertension 1988;12:585.
64. Dimsdale JE, Graham RM, Ziegler MG, et al. Age, race, diagnosis, and sodium effects on the pressor response to infused norepinephrine. Hypertension 1987;10:564.
65. Feinleib M, Garrison R, Borhani N, et al. Studies of Hypertension in Twins. In O Paul (ed), Epidemiology and Control of Hypertension. New York: Stratton International Medical, 1975;3.
66. Feinleib M. Genetics and Familial Aggregation of Blood Pressure. Presented at the Fifth Hahneman International Symposium on Hypertension. San Juan, PR: January 1977.

67. Munger RG, Prineas RJ, Gomez-Marin O. Persistent elevation of blood pressure among children with a family history of hypertension: the Minneapolis Children's Blood Pressure Study. J Hypertens 1988;6:647.
68. Paterson TL, Kaplan RM, Sallis JF, Nader PR. Aggregation of blood pressure in Anglo-American and Mexican-American families. Prev Med 1987;16:616.
69. Perusse L, Rice T, Bouchard C, et al. Cardiovascular risk factors in a French-Canadian population: resolution of genetic and familial environmental effects on blood pressure by using extensive information on environmental correlates. Am J Hum Genet 1989;45:240.
70. Miyao S, Furusho T. Genetic study of essential hypertension. Jpn Circ J 1978;42:1161.
71. Burke GL, Voors AW, Shear CL, et al. Blood pressure. Pediatrics 1987;80:784.
72. Clarke WR, Schrott HG, Leaverton PE, et al. Tracking of blood lipids and blood pressures in school age children: the Muscatine Study. Circulation 1978;58:626.
73. Voors AW, Webber LS, Berenson GS. Time course study of blood pressure in children over a three-year period—Bogalusa Heart Study. Hypertension 1980;2:102.
74. Higgins MW, Keller JB, Metzner HL, et al. Studies of blood pressure in Tecumseh, Michigan. II. Antecedents in childhood of high blood pressure in young adults. Hypertension 1980;2:117.
75. Woynarowska B, Mukherjee D, Roche AF, Siervogel RM. Blood pressure changes during adolescence and subsequent adult blood pressure level. Hypertension 1985;7:695.
76. Gillman MW, Cook NR, Rosner B, et al. Identifying children at risk for development of essential hypertension. J Pediatr 1993;122:837.

CHAPTER 3

Causes of Hypertension in Children

Leonard G. Feld and Patricia A. Veiga

Childhood hypertension has many diverse etiologies. It is useful to categorize the causes as either primary or secondary. Primary, or essential, hypertension is not caused by an identifiable abnormality and is most common in older children and adolescents. The causes of essential hypertension include hereditary, dietary, and environmental factors. Hypertension in newborns and young children is called secondary hypertension, or hypertension due to a specific and potentially correctable cause. A full list of these causes is presented in Table 3.4. Neonatal hypertension is primarily due to vascular, renal, endocrine, or drug-related causes. The etiology of secondary hypertension in the infant and child is extensive.

Essential Hypertension

Essential hypertension is the leading cause of high blood pressure (BP) in older children and adults. It is difficult to identify the specific cause of this form of hypertension, because of the heterogeneous nature of the disorder. Because hypertension is a significant risk factor in the development of premature cardiovascular morbidity and mortality, it is beneficial to identify elevated BP in children. Risk factors for the development of essential hypertension, which are identified in the adult population, should also be examined in children (Table 3.1).

Hereditary and Environmental Factors

It is well established that essential hypertension aggregates in families, suggesting a hereditary role in the transmission of hypertension [1]. These

TABLE 3.1
Factors Involved in the Development of Essential Hypertension

---

Heredity
Sodium intake
Chloride intake
Potassium intake
Calcium intake
Magnesium intake
Uric acid metabolism
Hyperinsulinemia/insulin resistance
Sodium-lithium countertransport
Red blood cell sodium content
Renal kallikrein-kinin and prostaglandin systems
Renin-angiotensin system
Exercise
Intrauterine growth retardation

---

aggregates also reflect the common environmental factors shared by a family. Genetic factors have been established by studies examining the higher BP correlation in monozygotic than dizygotic twins [2]. Efforts to isolate genetic and environmental factors have involved the examination of adopted children [1]. In such studies, nonfamilial factors such as measurement error, physiologic variability, and environment had a significant impact on BP. Overall, children of hypertensive parents appear to be more at risk of developing high BP than children of normotensive parents [2, 3].

Diet

Diet is a prominent environmental factor associated with BP. It could be a safe and effective method of controlling hypertension in children, although studies of its efficacy in childhood are limited [4]. Sodium has been examined more than any other dietary electrolyte. High-salt diets have been shown to increase BP in some individuals [5]. Further study shows that only sodium chloride has an effect on BP, although many individuals are resistant to its hypertension-inducing effect. There can be genetic variability in the renin-angiotensin-aldosterone system that also influences BP and explains this resistance to sodium [6]. However, a study of newborn infants that compared normal and low sodium (one-third the sodium content of the normal diet) diets revealed that sodium intake is related to systolic BP even early in life [7].

Potassium intake has been shown to be inversely related to BP. Hypokalemia may have vasoconstrictive effects related to the sodium-potassium adenosinetriphosphatase (ATPase) channel on smooth muscle cells [8]. This vasoconstriction can induce sodium retention and volume expansion, thereby increasing BP [9]. Vasoconstriction may also be related to decreased urinary excretion of kallikrein (an enzyme involved in the formation of bradykinin, a vasodilator) [8]. Potassium supplementation has been shown to decrease BP in individuals with sodium-sensitive hypertension [10] (though Miller and colleagues did not observe any affect on BP from modest doses of supplemental potassium in normotensive children [11]). Therefore, salt-sensitive hypertensive children may benefit from a higher potassium–lower sodium diet. This diet will increase the urinary potassium-sodium ratio, which is believed to be the key to potassium-related control of BP [12].

There is also an inverse relationship between dietary calcium and BP. Studies of hypertensive adults have shown that a low intake of calcium is associated with the development of hypertension [13]. Parathyroid hormone levels are also higher in these individuals due to increased renal excretion of calcium. It is thought that abnormal calcium handling by vascular smooth muscle cells causes increased peripheral resistance and ultimately increased BP [13]. These muscle cells have raised intracellular calcium levels that increase smooth muscle tone and can relate to increased renin release, synthesis of norepinephrine, and stimulation of the sympathetic nervous system, all of which lead to increased BP [13, 14].

Magnesium intake may also be inversely related to BP. Although studies in children are lacking, a study of maternal prenatal diets found that the intake of potassium, calcium, and magnesium was inversely related to infant BP in the first year of life [15]. It appears that the prenatal cation intake is transported across the placenta and affects BP regulation in the fetus. This study suggests that dietary factors in pregnancy and early life could protect against the development of elevated BP later in life [15].

The above dietary factors that contribute to hypertension suggest that nonpharmacologic dietary therapy may be possible for children with increased BP (see Chapter 5).

Correlating Factors

Abnormal uric acid metabolism occurs in essential hypertension. Prebis and colleagues found hyperuricemia in 13 of 31 children with essential hypertension [16]. Twenty-four–hour urine collections in these children showed that the hyperuricemia was caused by decreased urate clearance. Hyperuricemia may contribute to or serve as a marker for the development of hypertension [16].

Essential hypertension has also been associated with abnormal carbohydrate metabolism. Hyperinsulinemia and insulin resistance (impaired insulin action on target tissues) occur in nonobese subjects and correlate with the severity of hypertension [17]. Potential effects of hyperinsulinemia that lead to hypertension include decreased renal sodium excretion and increased circulating catecholamine levels [18]. Conversely, hypertension may impair insulin's action on glucose metabolism through altered vascular resistance [18]. Rocchini and colleagues have shown that hyperinsulinemia may also be responsible for the salt-sensitive hypertension observed in obese adolescents [19]. The effects of weight loss on insulin and BP regulation in obese adolescents have been examined. Results suggest that weight loss due to both dietary changes and physical training bring about a significant decrease in both BP and fasting insulin levels [20].

Reports have focused on the relationship between BP and intracellular ion transport. In particular, sodium-lithium countertransport and erythrocyte sodium content have been studied. Red blood cells (RBCs) have been chosen for these investigations because these easily accessible cells share the metabolic abnormalities of cells (i.e., kidney, smooth muscle) involved in BP regulation, which have limited accessibility [21]. Increased intracellular sodium is thought to raise BP by increasing peripheral vascular resistance. Sodium-lithium countertransport and RBC sodium appear to be influenced by gender, race, body size, and family history of hypertension, as well as levels of alcohol, uric acid, serum lipids, and potassium [21]. A study of sodium-lithium countertransport in erythrocytes of children showed a significant elevation of this measurement in hypertensive children when compared to normotensive children [22]. Trevisan and co-authors found that male patients have both higher countertransport rates and higher sodium concentration of RBCs than female patients [23]. In this study of 417 children and adults, blacks had a higher RBC sodium concentration but a lower rate of sodium-lithium countertransport than whites (Table 3.2). Therefore, intracellular sodium concentration alone does not determine countertransport. A later study examined countertransport rates and sodium content of RBCs in 311 sixth-grade children [24]. The family history of hypertension did not predict RBC sodium content or sodium-lithium countertransport rates. Factors such as lipids and body size also influence cation transport. Sodium-lithium countertransport correlates with weight, but has an inverse relationship to high density lipoprotein cholesterol [25]. In summary, the cellular handling of sodium appears to influence BP. Although limited data are available from studies in children, RBC cation transport may provide a useful screening tool for children and young adults predisposed to essential hypertension. Identifying these children allows the practitioner to strongly encourage the healthy habits of diet, exercise, and reasonable body weight, which can determine adult BP [21].

Both the renal kallikrein-kinin and prostaglandin systems play a role in BP regulation. Kallikrein is a peptidase produced in the kidney that generates bradykinin from kininogen. Kinins increase renal blood flow and decrease tubular reabsorption of sodium (Figure 3.1) [26]. Thus, the renal kallikrein-kinin system influences BP by promoting vasodilation and natriuresis. Urinary kallikrein activity was found to be significantly lower in grade school children with higher BPs [27, 28]. Urinary kallikrein excretion is highly hereditary and may be useful for predicting, at an early age, children at an increased risk for developing essential hypertension [29].

TABLE 3.2
Sodium-Lithium Countertransport and Red Cell Sodium Concentration by Sex
and Race

Sex	Race	
	White (n)	Black (n)
Sodium-lithium countertransport (μmol/liter red blood cell/min)		
Men	5.38 ± 1.94 (229)	3.91 ± 1.27 (33)
Women	4.36 ± 1.47 (97)	3.47 ± 1.49 (58)
Red cell sodium concentration (mmol/liter red blood cell)		
Men	6.69 ± 1.15 (229)	8.36 ± 2.07 (33)
Women	6.33 ± 1.23 (97)	7.92 ± 2.26 (58)

Source: Reproduced with permission from M Trevisan, D Ostrow, RS Cooper, et al. Sex and
race differences in sodium-lithium countertransport and red cell sodium concentration. Am J
Epidemiol 1984;120:539.

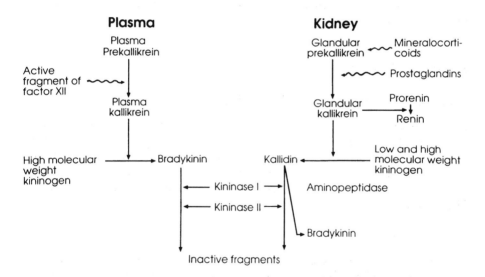

FIGURE 3.1. Renal kallikrein-kinin system. (Reproduced with permission from B
Waeber, J Nussberger, HR Brunner. In JH Laragh, BM Brenner [eds], Hypertension:
Pathophysiology, Diagnosis, and Management. New York: Raven, 1990;2214.)

On the other hand, the role of renal prostaglandins in regulating BP
is not clear, but it appears to be related to the renal kallikrein-kinin system. Kinins within the kidney promote the synthesis of renal
prostaglandins. These prostaglandins augment the vasodilator-diuretic
action of the kallikrein-kinin system [30, 31]. Activity of the renal
prostaglandin system has been studied by measuring urinary
prostaglandin excretion rates. Prostaglandin levels in the urine reflect

intrarenal synthesis [32]. It is known that renal prostaglandin $F_{2\alpha}$ excretion increases and prostaglandin E_2 excretion decreases with gestational age, and that both of these correlate with the normal rise in BP from preterm to term infant [33]. In adults with essential hypertension, urinary prostaglandin (PGE_2) excretion is decreased and may reflect an inadequate adaptive response to vasoconstrictor stimuli [32]. However, such studies in children with essential hypertension are not available.

Finally, low birth weight may be tied to the development of hypertension. Gennser and colleagues studied 104 male army recruits and found that the risk of high diastolic BP was significantly higher among men who had been growth retarded at birth. They suggested that intrauterine growth retardation may be a predictor of increased BP in early adult life [34]. Similarly, Barker and co-authors suggested that high placenta size could also predict increased risk of hypertension in adulthood [35]. Therefore it is useful to monitor both intrauterine growth rate and placenta size as possible warning signs for the future development of hypertension.

Secondary Hypertension

Secondary Hypertension in Neonates

Neonatal hypertension is now diagnosed frequently due to the improved methods of newborn BP monitoring and standardized values for BP measurements in newborn infants [36]. The reported causes include vascular causes, intrinsic renal disease, drugs, endocrine disease, abdominal and genitourinary surgery, pulmonary disease, and unknown causes (Table 3.3).

Renovascular Disease

The most common cause of secondary neonatal hypertension is renovascular disease. Thromboembolic complications from indwelling umbilical artery catheters have been recognized for many years as contributing to the increased incidence of hypertension in neonates [37, 38]. In such cases, hypertension is secondary to renin released by the viable, underperfused areas of the kidney. Prognosis for infants with thromboembolic complications is good with antihypertensive therapy, but persistent abnormalities in renal size and function can occur [39, 40]. After therapy, BP is normalized, but many of these infants still remain at risk of developing hypertension due to persistent renal changes [40].

Two other causes of renovascular hypertension in the neonate are renal artery stenosis (with or without the congenital rubella syndrome) and renal vein thrombosis [41]. The hypertension in these cases is renin dependent and increased plasma-renin levels are usually reported [42].

TABLE 3.3
Causes of Secondary Hypertension in the Newborn

Vascular
    Renal artery thrombosis
    Renal artery stenosis
    Renal vein thrombosis
    Aortic thrombosis
    Coarctation of the aorta
Kidney
    Acute renal failure
    Renal cortical/medullary necrosis
    Renal hypoplasia/dysplasia
    Renal tumors
    Obstructive uropathy
    Congenital nephrosis
    Autosomal recessive polycystic kidney disease
Medications
    Corticosteroids
    Ocular phenylephrine
    Narcotic-addicted mothers
    Cocaine
    Theophylline
    Pancuronium
Miscellaneous
    Fluid overload
    Increased intracranial pressure
    Pneumothorax
    Birth asphyxia
    Congenital adrenal hyperplasia
    Hyperaldosteronism
    Hypercalcemia
    Thyrotoxicosis
    Bronchopulmonary dysplasia
    Genitourinary tract surgery/omphalocele repair
    Extracorporeal membrane oxygenation
    Urinoma
    Adrenal hemorrhage
    Neuroblastoma
    Essential hypertension (rare)

Coarctation of the aorta can also cause hypertension. This vascular lesion causes hypertension in the newborn either due to a mechanical obstruction at the stenotic site or the vascular resistance of collateral vessels. In these cases, plasma renin and angiotensin II are elevated because of renal hypoperfusion. It is not clear if renal nerves and the sympathetic nervous system are also involved in this form of hypertension [43].

Renal Causes

Renal causes of neonatal hypertension include acute renal failure, renal cortical or medullary necrosis, renal hypoplasia, or renal dysplasia. In renal dysplasia, hypertension occurs due to poor renal perfusion to the more differentiated nephron units [44]. In acute renal necrosis, hypertension can also result from intravascular overload [45]. In congenital nephrosis, hypertension can be a physiologic response to decreased plasma volume. On the other hand, hypovolemia triggers angiotensin release and peripheral vasoconstriction to the extent that BP increases despite hypovolemia [46]. Renal tumors such as congenital mesoblastic nephroma are also associated with a high incidence of hypertension due to compression of the renal artery and increased renin activity [47]. Additionally, ureteropelvic junction obstruction can be associated with hypertension and is due to ischemia and high renin activity in the case of unilateral hydronephrosis or sodium and water retention with normal renins in the case of bilateral hydronephrosis (Figure 3.2) [48]. Renin-mediated hypertension is also frequent in autosomal recessive polycystic kidney disease [49].

Medications

Hypertension is also observed in association with various medications. Corticosteroids cause sodium and water retention, which leads to hypertension. [50]. BP is also increased by ocular 10% phenylephrine, which is readily absorbed and enters the circulation causing vasoconstriction [51]. Theophylline and cocaine (ingested via breast milk) increase norepinephrine levels by blocking its uptake at nerve terminals. Both are associated with neonatal hypertension [52].

Miscellaneous Causes

Another frequent cause of hypertension in neonates is fluid overload caused by excessive administration of blood products or crystalloid solutions (isotonic saline). Increased intracranial pressure and cerebrovascular accidents are associated with hypertension due to the disturbance of medullary vasomotor centers and the subsequent activation of the sympathetic nervous system. Elevated BP is detected in infants with pneumothorax and birth asphyxia. Shock and hypoxia stimulate the renin-angiotensin system due to renal hypoperfusion, and result in an increased release of catecholamines, renin, and antidiuretic hormones, which can lead to hypertension. Finally, decreased sodium and water excretion in neonates with renal insufficiency is a major contributing factor to hypertension due to salt and water overload. [53].

Endocrine causes of hypertension include congenital adrenal hyperplasia and hyperaldosteronism. In these cases, sodium retention, plasma volume expansion, and low plasma renin activity are the major factors in increasing systemic BP [54]. Hypercalcemia increases peripheral vascular

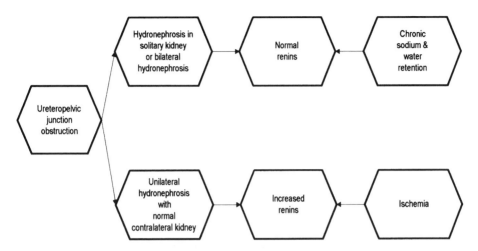

FIGURE 3.2. Mechanisms for hypertension in ureteropelvic junction obstruction. (Reproduced with permission from IC Grossman, WJ Cromie, AJ Wein, JW Duckett. Renal hypertension secondary to ureteropelvic junction obstruction. Unusual presentation and new therapeutic modality. Urology 1981;17:69.)

resistance through the adrenal release of epinephrine [55]. Hypertension in neonatal thyrotoxicosis is associated with a wide pulse pressure [56]. In neonatal thyrotoxicosis, the systolic BP rises to accommodate the increased cardiac output and stroke volume and the decreased systemic vascular resistance [57].

Bronchopulmonary dysplasia can be accompanied by hypertension due to vasoconstrictive mediators triggered by chronic lung disease. Hypoxia and hypercarbia increase systemic vascular resistance through the release of catecholamines and increased vasomotor tone [58]. In children with hypoxia and respiratory distress syndrome, elevated angiotensin-converting enzyme activity occurs [59]. Hypertension may also occur following both genitourinary tract surgery and closure of abdominal wall defects and is related to elevated renin activity and increased catecholamine release [60, 61].

Hypertension is also a common complication of extracorporeal membrane oxygenation (ECMO). Sell and co-authors found systolic hypertension in 38 of 41 newborns treated with ECMO [62]. Results of assays of biochemical mediators showed elevated renin and catecholamine levels. Expanded extracellular volume may also contribute to the development of hypertension in children treated with ECMO.

Transient renin-mediated hypertension secondary to renal artery or kidney compression or obstruction can be associated with urinoma and adrenal hemorrhage [63, 64]. Excess catecholamines also cause hypertension in congenital neuroblastoma.

Finally, primary hypertension or elevated BP can be a significant problem in the neonate following discharge from a neonatal intensive care unit. Such hypertension responds to medical therapy and therapy can ultimately be discontinued [65].

Secondary Hypertension in Infants and Children

Secondary hypertension in older infants and children also has many potential causes (Tables 3.4 and 3.5). Although the list is extensive, the most common causes of secondary hypertension in older children are obesity, coarctation of the aorta, and renal parenchymal and vascular disease.

Obesity

The incidence of obesity in children is increasing in the United States. Obesity is associated with many medical problems including elevated BP [66]. Excessive weight gain can be associated with the development of hypertension in adulthood [67]. Obesity elevates BP by expanding cardiac stroke volume in a mild volume overload state [68]. Insulin resistance and hyperinsulinemia may also lead to hypertension by increasing either renal sodium reabsorption or sympathetic nervous system activity [20].

Renal Causes

Renal causes of secondary hypertension are a consequence of salt and water retention and elevated plasma renin activity. Such causes include acute and chronic glomerulopathies, renal hypoplasia (kidneys that are too small for height or age), obstructive uropathy, and reflux nephropathy. Decreased salt and water excretion in chronic renal failure/insufficiency causes hypertension by expanding extracellular volume. Elevated BP can result from overactivity of the renin-angiotensin system, diminished baroreceptor sensitivity, enhanced sympathetic nervous system activity, or decreased secretion of vasodilating substances such as prostaglandins and kallikrein [69, 70].

There are a number of conditions that increase BP by increasing renin release. In obstructive uropathy, chronic pyelonephritis may cause renal parenchymal scars (areas of renal ischemia), which stimulate renin release [71]. Ureteropelvic obstruction and unilateral hydronephrosis also stimulate renin release. Pyeloplasty restores normotension in these cases [72]. Hypertension in cystic kidney disease is also related to renin overproduction [73, 74]. Multicystic kidneys generally have no excretory function or perfusion on radionuclide scans, although delayed imaging shows activity around cysts [75]. This finding suggests limited vascular flow occurs and the decreased renal perfusion results in hypertension due to renin production by the more differentiated renal units [44].

TABLE 3.4
Secondary Causes of Hypertension in Older Infants and Children

Obesity
Renal disease
  Acute and chronic glomerulopathies
  Acute glomerulonephritis
  Nephrotic syndrome
  Alport's syndrome
  Acute renal failure
  Renal cortical or medullary necrosis
  Hemolytic-uremic syndrome
  Henoch-Schönlein purpura
  Systemic lupus erythematosus
  Chronic renal failure and insufficiency
  Renal hypoplasia
  Obstructive uropathy
  Reflux nephropathy and chronic pyelonephritis
  Cystic kidney disease
  Nephropathy secondary to diabetes mellitus, sickle cell disease, or interstitial
    nephritis
  Post–renal trauma
  Renal infarction
  Post–renal transplant
Vascular disease
  Coarctation of the aorta
  Hypoplastic aorta
  Marfan's syndrome
  Crossed renal ectopia
  Subacute bacterial endocarditis
  Aortic valve insufficiency
  Fibromuscular dysplasia
  Neurofibromatosis
  William's syndrome
  Atherosclerosis (progeria, inborn error of lipid metabolism)
  Takayasu's arteritis/arteritis
  Renal artery stenosis/aneurysm/fistula
  Renal artery compression (secondary to tumor or hematoma)
  Aortic thrombosis
  Renal vein thrombosis
  Arteriovenous fistula
  Renal transplantation (rejection, drugs)
Endocrine
  Cushing's syndrome
  Idiopathic primary hyperaldosteronism
  Glucocorticoid remediable (dexamethasone-suppressible) hypertension
  Mineralocorticoid excess (congenital adrenal hyperplasia, 17α-hydroxylase and
    11 β-hydroxylase deficiencies, licorice ingestion)
  Hyperthyroidism

TABLE 3.4. *(continued)*

Liddle's syndrome
Hyperparathyroidism, hypercalcemia, vitamin D intoxication
Gordon's syndrome
Tumor
  Wilms' tumor
  Tuberous sclerosis
  Hemangiopericytoma (renin-secreting)
  Pheochromocytoma (isolated or associated with multiple endocrinopathy syndrome, neurofibromatosis, or von Hippel-Lindau disease)
  Neuroblastoma and related neurogenic tumors
  Ovarian tumor
  Conn's syndrome
Drugs and toxins (see Chapter 4)
  Oral contraceptive pills
  Corticosteroids and adrenocorticotropic hormone
  Sympathomimetics (nose or eye drops, "cold" or "flu" medications)
  Amphetamines
  Methylphenidate
  Imipramine
  Clonidine withdrawal
  Metoclopramide
  Cyclosporine
  Methotrexate
  Theophylline
  Nonsteroidal anti-inflammatory agents
  Cisplatin
  Recombinant human erythropoietin
  Recreational drugs
  Lead
  Mercury
  Scorpion envenomation
  Cigarette smoking
  Caffeine
Neurologic
  Increased intracranial pressure
  Head injury or stroke
  Guillain-Barré syndrome
  Autonomic dysreflexia (spinal cord damage)
  Posterior fossa lesions
  Neurofibromatosis
  Poliomyelitis
  Dysautonomia
Other
  Sleep apnea
  Traction-induced immobilization
  Severe burns
  Genitourinary tract surgery

Anemia (systolic)
Asphyxia
Pneumothorax
Ventilator therapy
Pregnancy
Intravascular volume overload
Pain, anxiety, or stress
Alpha$_1$ antitrypsin deficiency from liver transplantation
Asphyxiating thoracic dystrophy (Jeune syndrome)

Source: Adapted from LG Feld, JE Springate. Hypertension in children. Curr Prob Pediatr 1988;18:330.

TABLE 3.5
Causes of Hypertension by Underlying Factor

Coarctation of the aorta
Renin-dependent hypertension
   Renal vascular disease
   Renal parenchymal disease
   Renal tumor
   Hyperthyroidism
   Genitourinary surgery
   Unilateral hydronephrosis
   Mercury
   Oral contraceptive pills
Hypervolemia
   Acute renal failure
   Chronic renal failure
   Excess blood, plasma, or saline
   Bilateral ureteropelvic junction obstruction
   Lead
   Nonsteroidal anti-inflammatory agents
   Corticosteroids
Acute hypovolemia
   Nephrotic syndrome relapse
   Burns
   Renal, adrenal, and gastrointestinal salt loss
Catecholamine excess
   Pheochromocytoma
   Neuroblastoma
   Hypercalcemia
   Lead
   Cigarettes
   Traction-induced immobilization
   Increased sympathetic nervous system
      Guillain-Barré syndrome
      Poliomyelitis
      Dysautomia

TABLE 3.5. *(continued)*

Corticosteroid excess
  Congenital adrenal hyperplasia
  Conn's syndrome
  Cushing's syndrome
  Low-renin hypertensive states
  Cigarettes
Central nervous system disease
  Tumor
  Head injury
  Seizure
  Infection
Drug therapy
  Corticosteroids
  Sympathomimetics
  Oral contraceptive pills
Essential

Source: Reproduced with permission from MJ Dillion. Clinical Aspects of Hypertension. In MA Holliday, TM Barratt, RL Vernier (eds), Pediatric Nephrology. Baltimore: Williams & Wilkins, 1987;751; and LG Feld, JE Springate. Hypertension in children. Curr Prob Pediatr 1988;18:330.

Hypertension in diabetes nephropathy is related to expansion of the extracellular fluid volume, increased systemic vascular resistance, and reduction in baroreceptor sensitivity [76]. Paulsen and colleagues showed that teenagers and young adults with insulin-dependent diabetes mellitus had high plasma renin activity [77]. Plasma renin activity, in subjects who developed elevated urinary albumin excretion, also remained high. However, among those with clinical proteinuria or diabetic renal disease, renin and aldosterone levels are usually low despite the presence of hypertension.

Renin-mediated hypertension follows renal trauma or infarction. Hypertension occurs frequently after renal transplantation due to pre-existing native renal disease, use of steroids or cyclosporine, graft rejection, or transplant renal artery stenosis [69, 78, 79]. Patients with sickle cell disease usually have lower than normal BP due to increased sodium and water excretion [80]. However, some patients with sickle cell nephropathy have nephrotic syndrome and develop renal failure and hypertension [81].

Vascular Causes

Coarctation of the aorta and renovascular disease can also lead to hypertension. Because of the mechanical obstruction of aortic blood flow, coarctation of the aorta is associated with hypertension. It is also associated with increased renin and angiotensin II activity caused by decreased renal perfusion pressure [82] (Figure 3.3).

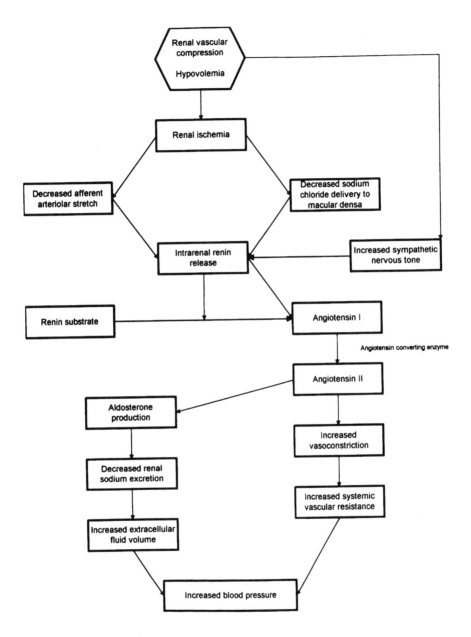

FIGURE 3.3. Renin-angiotensin system in renin-mediated hypertension. (Reproduced with permission from B Rose. Clinical Physiology of Acid-Base and Electrolyte Disorders [3rd ed]. New York: McGraw-Hill, 1989;46.)

Immediately following coarctation repair, hypertension is caused by excessive sympathetic nervous system activity and renin-angiotensin system activity [43]. In long-term follow-up, BP relates to primary baroreceptor alteration, or structural changes in the arterial wall, or both [83]. Renin-mediated hypertension occurs in patients with hypoplastic aorta, and in children with crossed renal ectopia [84]. Marfan's syndrome is also associated with hypertension because of chronic pyelonephritis and renal scarring [85]. Hypertension is an infrequent finding in subacute bacterial endocarditis, although hypertension may occur due to sodium and water retention [86]. In chronic aortic valve insufficiency, high systolic BP associated with a wide pulse pressure reflects a compensatory mechanism of increased sympathetic nervous system activity and catecholamine release [87].

Renovascular disease with hypertension includes fibromuscular dysplasia. This nonatherosclerotic and noninflammatory vascular disease most commonly involves the renal and carotid arteries, causing renovascular hypertension [88]. In adults with neurofibromatosis, hypertension is usually caused by a pheochromocytoma, whereas in children renal artery stenosis is more frequently the cause [89]. Peripheral vascular abnormalities (renal artery stenosis, long segmental narrowing of the aorta, and discrete coarctation of the aorta) in William's syndrome may also cause severe hypertension [90].

Other causes of renovascular hypertension include premature atherosclerosis, renal artery arteritis, renal artery stenosis, and renal artery calcification [91–95]. Renin-mediated hypertension is also observed in patients with renal arteriovenous fistula, renal artery compression, aortic thrombosis, or renal vein thrombosis [96, 97].

Endocrine Causes

Hypertension is common with several endocrine disorders. A wide pulse pressure and increased sympathetic nervous system activity are hallmarks of hyperthyroidism. In such cases, increased systolic BP reflects the inability of the vascular tree to accommodate the marked increase in cardiac output and stroke volume [57]. Catecholamine levels are normal but plasma renin activity is increased [98, 99]. Hyperparathyroidism and hypercalcemia heighten peripheral vascular resistance either by increasing adrenal release of epinephrine or as a direct effect of calcium on blood vessels [55]. Adrenocortical disorders increase systemic BP due to sodium and water retention. This increase in systemic BP is observed in Cushing's syndrome, congenital adrenal hyperplasia, idiopathic primary hyperaldosteronism, and apparent mineralocorticoid excess states [100–102].

Because of its sodium-retaining ingredient glycyrrhetinic acid, excessive licorice ingestion causes a mineralocorticoid excess state [101]. Long-term licorice ingestion inhibits 11β-hydroxysteroid dehydrogenase activity and impairs cortisol metabolism [103]. Excessive sodium reabsorption occurs

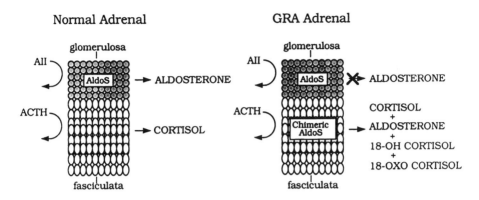

FIGURE 3.4. Adrenal abnormality in glucocorticoid-remediable aldosteronism (GRA). Left panel: the normal adrenal gland. Right panel: the chimeric aldosterone synthase production from the fasciculata. (Reproduced with permission from RP Lifton, RG Dluhy, M Powers, et al. Hereditary hypertension caused by chimaeric gene duplications and ectopic expression of aldosterone synthase. Nat Genet 1992;2:66.)

in Gordon's syndrome, which is characterized by severe hyperkalemia, suppressed renin and aldosterone, and hypertension that can be reversed by sodium restriction [104]. Glucocorticoid-remediable aldosteronism (GRA) is an autosomal dominant form of hypertension and is the result of chimeric gene duplications arising from unequal crossing-over of regulatory sequences of steroid 11β-hydroxylase with coding sequences of aldosterone synthase (Figure 3.4) [105]. This regulatory mutation results in the ectopic expression of the aldosterone synthase activity that is under the control of adrenocorticotropic hormone (ACTH). This abnormality causes elevated plasma aldosterone concentration, suppressed plasma renin activity, and high urinary levels of abnormal adrenal steroids (18-hydroxycortisol and 18-oxocortisol).

Tumors

Both renal and extra-renal tumors cause hypertension. Renal tumors include Wilms' tumor, which secretes renin or compresses the renal artery, thereby leading to ischemic hyper-reninism [106, 107]. Hemangiopericytoma is a rare renin-secreting juxtaglomerular cell tumor, which is associated with severe hypertension and hypokalemic alkalosis [104, 108, 109]. Hypertension in tuberous sclerosis may be secondary to renal hamartoma formation with primary reninism [110].

Extra-renal tumors include pheochromocytoma, which is a rare pediatric tumor arising from the sympathoadrenal system and secreting primarily catecholamines [111]. Clinical signs include unusually labile BP, paroxysms of hypertension, and spells of perspiration, tachycardia, and headache [112]. After surgical removal of the tumor, follow-up is essential because a recurrent tumor may appear several years later. Return of the tumor is marked by recurrent symptoms and signs of hypertension [113]. Another rare pediatric tumor, aldosterone-secreting adenoma (Conn's syndrome), is also associated with hypertension, elevated aldosterone, and suppressed plasma renin activity [114]. Hypertension also occurs with neurogenic tumors such as neuroblastoma and ganglioneuroma because of excessive circulating catecholamines, hyper-reninism due to renal artery compression, or elevated cortisol levels [115].

Drugs and Toxins

Hypertension has been reported with a variety of drugs and toxins (see Chapter 4). Oral contraceptive pills raise plasma renin activity by increasing estrogen-induced renin substrate [116]. Saruta and colleagues suggested that in certain individuals, BP rises inappropriately due to a diminished feedback suppression of renin release despite increased renin substrate. Pre-existing hypertension may also be intensified by oral contraceptives [117]. Likewise, the use of ACTH hormones in children with infantile spasms results in hypertension secondary to a hyperglucocorticoid state (excess sodium and water retention) [118]. Transient hypertension with use of intravenous antidopaminergic drugs (such as metaclopramide) may be related to catecholamine release [119–121]. Additionally, nasal phenylephrine and oral pseudoephrine cause hypertension through vasoconstriction [122]. Rebound hypertension occurs with clonidine withdrawal due to increased plasma catecholamines or hypersensitivity to alpha-adrenergic receptor stimulation [123]. Due to its nephrotoxic effects (altered intrarenal prostaglandin synthesis and altered intrarenal hemodynamic function), cyclosporine use in transplant recipients is also a frequent cause of hypertension [124]. Nonsteroidal anti-inflammatory agents also raise BP (rarely) by increasing vascular resistance and fluid retention [31]. Intra-arterial cisplatin is associated with persistent hypertension secondary to renal vascular toxicity [125]. Furthermore, recombinant erythropoietin replacement therapy in children with end-stage renal disease accelerates pre-existing high BP [126]. This may be due to a rapid rise in hematocrit. More likely it is the increase in blood viscosity or decrease in hypoxic vasodilation which unmasks or aggravates BP in the chronic renal failure patient prone to hypertension [127].

Lead intoxication causes hypertension by vasoconstriction, sodium and water retention, low plasma renin activity, and increased central and peripheral sympathetic nervous system activity [128]. Likewise, toxins such as mercury and scorpion envenomation result in hypertension due to excess catecholamines and plasma renin activity [129, 130]. Cigarette smoking raises plasma aldosterone, cortisol, and catecholamine levels resulting in increased heart rate and hypertension [131]. Caffeine intake increases BP but not on a long-term basis. The origin of caffeine's pressor effect is unclear [132].

Neurologic Causes

Hypertension is common in several neurologic disorders. Head injury and increased intracranial pressure (due to tumor, hematoma, or meningitis) may lead to both abnormal cerebral regulation and reflex activation of the sympathetic nervous system resulting in elevated systolic BP and increased circulating catecholamines [133, 134]. In Guillain-Barré syndrome, excessive sympathetic activity is also the result of autonomic dysfunction, and wide fluctuations of BP from severe hypertension to hypotension are observed [135]. Autonomic dysreflexia in a patient with a spinal cord injury can result in hypertension. This hypertension is secondary to increased reflex activity within the nervous system and is usually triggered by a noxious stimuli below the level of the injury [136]. Disturbance of the medullary vasomotor center also causes hypertension in poliomyelitis and dysautonomia [40].

Miscellaneous Causes

Several other medical conditions can lead to secondary hypertension. In severe burns, extracellular fluid depletion causes vasoconstriction and a massive release of angiotensin. Genitourinary tract surgery releases renin, which also leads to increased BP. Because anemia is a hyperdynamic state, systolic hypertension results from the attempt to accommodate the abnormal decrease in peripheral vascular resistance and the increase in cardiac output due to hypoxia [137]. Asphyxia and pneumothorax with shock and hypoxia elevate BP through activation of the renin-angiotensin system. In addition to increasing intrathoracic pressure, and decreasing cardiac output and renal perfusion, ventilator therapy may also alter intrarenal blood flow. This alteration contributes to increased renin and vasopressin levels, as well as decreased urinary sodium excretion [138]. Hypertension is also reported in association with reflex adrenergic activity, which is a result of sleep apnea (Figure 3.5). Likewise, chronic hypercapnia, hypoxia, and acidosis may stimulate reflex arteriolar constriction and therefore increase BP [139].

Elevated plasma renin activity is one of several complications that cause traction-induced hypertension. [140]. Traction may stretch sympathetic nerves around blood vessels causing vasoconstriction [141]. The prolonged bed rest also promotes renal salt and water retention [142]. In addition, immobilization hypercalcemia increases both vascular tone and BP [141].

Pregnancy-induced hypertension is thought to result from placental ischemia and an increase in peripheral vascular resistance [143]. This altered vascular reactivity may relate to decreased vasodilating prostaglandins [144]. However, stress, anxiety, and pain also produce

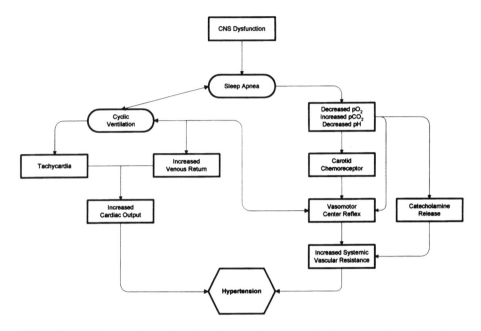

FIGURE 3.5. Proposed mechanism for cyclic systemic hypertension with sleep apnea that may lead to sustained hypertension. (Reproduced with permission from US Schroeder, J Mott, C Guilleminault. Sleep Apnea Syndromes. New York: Alan R. Liss, 1978;191.)

changes in cardiac stroke volume and total peripheral vascular resistance in selected individuals [145].

Children with alpha$_1$ antitrypsin deficiency and liver transplants frequently display hypertension attributed to cyclosporine toxicity, but these children also have a higher incidence of pre-operative glomerulonephritis [146]. Jeune's syndrome (asphyxiating thoracic dystrophy) may also involve the kidneys and result in chronic renal failure and hypertension [147].

References

1. Mongeau J-G. Heredity and blood pressure in humans: an overview. Pediatr Nephrol 1987;1:69.
2. Mongeau J-G. Heredity and blood pressure. Semin Nephrol 1989;9:208.
3. Shear CL, Burke GL, Freedman DS, Berenson GS. Value of childhood blood pressure measurements and family history in predicting future blood pressure status: results from 8 years of follow up in the Bogalusa heart study. Pediatrics 1986;77:862.
4. Grobbee DE. Diet and blood pressure. Semin Nephrol 1989;9:222.

5. Luft FC. Sodium: complexities in a simple relationship. Hosp Pract (Off Ed) 1988;23:73.
6. Weinberger MH. Dietary sodium and blood pressure. Hosp Pract (Off Ed) 1986;21:55.
7. Hofman A, Hazebroek A, Valkenburg HA. A randomized trial of sodium intake and blood pressure in newborn infants. JAMA 1983;250:370.
8. Svetkey LP, Klotman PE. Blood Pressure and Potassium Intake. In JH Laragh, BM Brenner (eds), Hypertension: Pathophysiology, Diagnosis, and Management. New York: Raven, 1990;217.
9. Krishna GG. Effect of potassium intake on blood pressure. J Am Soc Nephrol 1990;1:43.
10. Linas SL. The role of potassium in the pathogenesis and treatment of hypertension. Kidney Int 1991;39:771.
11. Miller JZ, Weinberger MH, Christian JC. Blood pressure response to potassium supplementation in normotensive adults and children. Hypertension 1987;10:437.
12. Sinaiko AR. General Consideration and Clinical Approach to the Management. In JMH Loggie (ed), Pediatric and Adolescent Hypertension. Boston: Blackwell, 1992;119.
13. McCarron DA. Calcium: confirming an inverse relationship. Hosp Pract (Off Ed) 1989;24:137.
14. Gruskin AB, Dabbagh S, Fleischmann LE. Mechanisms of Hypertension in Childhood Disease. In MA Holliday, TM Barratt, ED Avner (eds), Pediatric Nephrology (3rd ed). Baltimore: Williams & Wilkins, 1994;1096.
15. McGarvey ST, Zinner SH, Willet WC, Rosner B. Maternal prenatal dietary potassium, calcium, magnesium, and infant blood pressure. Hypertension 1991;17:218.
16. Prebis JW, Gruskin AB, Polinsky MS, Baluarte HJ. Uric acid in childhood essential hypertension. J Pediatr 1981;98:702.
17. Ferrannini E, Buzzigoli G, Bonadonna R, et al. Insulin resistance in essential hypertension. N Engl J Med 1987;317:350.
18. Buchanan T. Insulin resistance and hyperinsulinemia: implications for the pathogenesis and treatment of hypertension. Semin Nephrol 1991;11:512.
19. Rocchini AP. Insulin resistance and blood pressure regulation in obese and nonobese subjects. Hypertension 1991;17:837.
20. Rocchini AP, Katch V, Schork A, Kelch RP. Insulin and blood pressure during weight loss in obese adolescents. Hypertension 1987;10:267.
21. Trevisan M, Krogh V, Dorn J, DeSanto NG. Blood pressure and intracellular ion transport in childhood. Semin Nephrol 1989;9:253.
22. Norling LL, Landt M, Goldring D, et al. Lithium-sodium (Li-Na) countertransport (CT) in erythrocytes of children with hypertension (HPT). Pediatr Res 1982;16:104.
23. Trevisan M, Ostrow D, Cooper RS, et al. Sex and race differences in sodium-lithium countertransport and red cell sodium concentration. Am J Epidemiol 1984;120:537.
24. Trevisan M, Strazzullo P, Cappuccio FP, et al. Red blood cell Na content, Na, Li-countertransport, family history of hypertension and blood pressure in school children. J Hypertens 1988;6:227.
25. Hunt SC, Williams RR, Smith JB, Ash KO. Association of three erythrocyte cation transport systems with plasma lipids in Utah subjects. Hypertension 1986;8:30.

26. Haycock G. Sodium and Water. In MA Holliday, TM Barratt, RL Vernier (eds), Pediatric Nephrology. Baltimore: Williams & Wilkins, 1987;81.
27. Sinaiko AR, Glasser RJ, Gillum RF, Prineas RJ. Urinary kallikrein excretion in grade school children with high and low blood pressure. J Pediatr 1982;100:938.
28. McGarvey ST, Zinner SH, Margolius HS, et al. Urinary kallikrein (UKal) reproducibility and relation to blood pressure [BP] in young children. Circulation 1986;74(Suppl II):488.
29. Berry TD, Hasstedt SJ, Hunt SC, et al. A gene for high urinary kallikrein may protect against hypertension in Utah kindreds. Hypertension 1989;13:3.
30. Nasjletti A, Malik KU. The renal kallikrein-kinin and prostaglandin systems interaction. Annu Rev Physiol 1981;43:597.
31. Quilley J, Quilley CP, McGiff JC. Eicosanoids and Hypertension. In JH Laragh, BM Brenner (eds), Hypertension: Pathophysiology, Diagnosis, and Management. New York: Raven, 1990;829.
32. Cinotti GA, Pugliese F. Prostaglandins and blood pressure regulation. Kidney Int 1988;34:57.
33. Robillard JE. The Roles of Kallikrein-Kinin and Prostaglandin Systems in Juvenile Essential Hypertension. In JMH Loggie, MJ Horan, AR Hohn, et al (eds), Proceedings of the NHLBI Workshop on Juvenile Hypertension. New York: Biomedical Information Corporation, 1984;231.
34. Gennser G, Rymark P, Isberg PE. Low birth weight and risk of high blood pressure in adulthood. Br Med J 1988;296:1498.
35. Barker DJP, Bull AR, Osmond C, Simmonds SJ. Fetal and placental size and risk of hypertension in adult life. Br Med J 1990;301:259.
36. Tan KL. Blood pressure in full-term healthy neonates. Clin Pediatr (Phila) 1987;26:21.
37. Plumer LB, Kaplan GW, Mendoza SA. Hypertension in infants—a complication of umbilical arterial catheterization. J Pediatr 1976;89:802.
38. Baldwin CE, Holder TM, Ashcraft KW, Amoury RA. Neonatal renovascular hypertension—a complication of aortic monitoring catheters. J Pediatr Surg 1981;16:820.
39. Caplan MS, Cohn RA, Langman CB, et al. Favorable outcome of neonatal aortic thrombosis and renovascular hypertension. J Pediatr 1989;115:291.
40. Adelman RD. Long-term follow-up of neonatal renovascular hypertension. Pediatr Nephrol 1987;1:35.
41. Menser MA, Dorman DC, Reye RDK, Reid RR. Renal-artery stenosis in the rubella syndrome. Lancet 1966;1:790.
42. Angella JJ, Sommer LS, Poole C, Fogel BJ. Neonatal hypertension associated with renal artery hypoplasia. Pediatrics 1968;41:524.
43. Bagby SB. Dissection of Pathogenetic Factors in Coarctation Hypertension. In JMH Loggie, MJ Horan, AR Hohn, et al (eds), Presented at the NHLBI Workshop on Juvenile Hypertension. New York: Biomedical Information Corporation, 1984;253.
44. Chen YH, Stapleton FB, Roy S, Noe HN. Neonatal hypertension from a unilateral multicystic dysplastic kidney. J Urol 1985;133:664.
45. Anand SK, Northway JD, Smith JA. Neonatal renal papillary and cortical necrosis. Am J Dis Child 1977;131:773.

46. Dillion MJ. Clinical Aspects of Hypertension. In MA Holliday, TM Barratt, RL Vernier (eds), Pediatric Nephrology. Baltimore: Williams & Wilkins, 1987;743.
47. Chan HSL, Cheng M-Y, Mancer K, et al. Congenital mesoblastic nephroma: a clinicoradiologic study of 17 cases representing the pathologic spectrum of the disease. J Pediatr 1987;111:64.
48. Grossman IC, Cromie WJ, Wein AJ, Duckett JW. Renal hypertension secondary to ureteropelvic junction obstruction. Unusual presentation and new therapeutic modality. Urology 1981;17:69.
49. Cole BR, Conley SB, Stapleton FB. Polycystic kidney disease in the first year of life. J Pediatr 1987;111:693.
50. Kazzi NJ, Brans YW, Poland RL. Dexamethasone effects on the hospital course of infants with bronchopulmonary dysplasia who are dependent on artificial ventilation. Pediatrics 1990;86:722.
51. Isenberg S, Everett S. Cardiovascular effects of mydriatics in low–birth-weight infants. J Pediatr 1984;105:111.
52. Chasnoff IJ, Lewis DE, Squires L. Cocaine intoxication in a breast-fed infant. Pediatrics 1987;80:836.
53. Guignard J-P. Neonatal Nephrology. In MA Holliday, TM Barratt, RL Vernier (eds), Pediatric Nephrology. Baltimore: Williams & Wilkins, 1987;921.
54. Bongiovanni AM. Renin activity, aldosterone secretion, and congenital adrenal hyperplasia. Pediatrics 1968;41:871.
55. Marone C, Beretta-Piccoli C, Weidmann P. Acute hypercalcemic hypertension in man: role of hemodynamics, catecholamines, and renin. Kidney Int 1980;20:92.
56. Eason E, Costom B, Papageorgiou AN. Hypertension in neonatal thyrotoxicosis. J Pediatr 1982;100:766.
57. Klein I. Thyroid Hormone and Blood Pressure Regulation. In JH Laragh, BM Brenner (eds), Hypertension: Pathophysiology, Diagnosis, and Management. New York: Raven, 1990;1661.
58. Abman SH, Warady BA, Lum GM, Koops BL. Systemic hypertension in infants with bronchopulmonary dysplasia. J Pediatr 1984;104:929.
59. Mattioli L, Zakheim RM, Mullis K, Molteni A. Angiotensin-I–converting enzyme activity in idiopathic respiratory distress syndrome of the newborn infant and in experimental alveolar hypoxia in mice. J Pediatr 1975;87:97.
60. Gilboa N, Urizar RE. Severe hypertension in newborn after pyeloplasty of hydronephrotic kidney. Urology 1983;22:179.
61. Adelman RD, Sherman MP. Hypertension in the neonate following closure of abdominal wall defects. J Pediatr 1980;97:642.
62. Sell LL, Cullen ML, Lerner GR, et al. Hypertension during extracorporeal membrane oxygenation: cause, effect, and management. Surgery 1987;102:724.
63. Sirinelli D, Biriotti V, Schmit P, et al. Urinoma and arterial hypertension complicating neonatal renal candidiasis. Pediatr Radiol 1987;17:156.
64. Sirota L, Strauss S, Rechnitz Y, et al. Transient obstruction of the kidney and hypertension due to neonatal adrenal hemorrhage. Helv Paediat Acta 1985;40:177.
65. Friedman AL, Hustead VA. Hypertension in babies following discharge from a neonatal intensive care unit. Pediatr Nephrol 1987;1:30.
66. Unger R, Kreeger L, Christoff KK. Childhood obesity. Medical and familial correlates and age of onset. Clin Pediatr (Phila) 1990;29:368.

67. Havlik RJ, Hubert HB, Fabsitz RR, Feinleib M. Weight and hypertension. Ann Intern Med 1983;98:855.
68. Messerli FH. Obesity in hypertension: how innocent a bystander? Am J Med 1984;77:1077.
69. Balfe JW, Levin L, Tsuru N, Chan JCM. Hypertension in childhood. Adv Pediatr 1989;36:201.
70. Acosta JH. Hypertension in chronic renal disease. Kidney Int 1982;22:702.
71. Munoz AL, Pascual y Baralt JF, Melendez MT. Arterial hypertension in infants with hydronephrosis. Report of six cases. Am J Dis Child 1977;131:38.
72. Carella JA, Silber I. Hyperreninemic hypertension in an infant secondary to pelviureteric obstruction treated successfully by surgery. J Pediatr 1976;88:987.
73. Bennett WM, Elzinga LW, Barry JM. Polycystic kidney disease: II. Diagnosis and management. Hosp Pract (Off Ed) 1992;27:59.
74. Susskind MR, Kim KS, King LR. Hypertension and multicystic kidney. Urology 1989;34:362.
75. Warshawsky AB, Miller KE, Kaplan GW. Urographic visualization of multicystic kidneys. J Urol 1977;117:94.
76. Sower JR, Levy J, Zemel MB. Hypertension and diabetes. Med Clin North Am 1988;72:1399.
77. Paulsen EP, Seip RL, Ayers CR, et al. Plasma renin activity and albumin excretion in teenage type I diabetic subjects. A prospective study. Hypertension 1989;13:781.
78. Broyer M, Guest G, Gagnadoux MF, Beurton D. Hypertension following renal transplantation in children. Pediatr Nephrol 1987;1:16.
79. Sinaiko AR, Wells TG. Childhood Hypertension. In JH Laragh, BM Brenner (eds), Hypertension: Pathophysiology, Diagnosis, and Management. New York: Raven, 1990;1853.
80. Johnson CS, Giorgio AJ. Arterial blood pressure in adults with sickle cell disease. Arch Intern Med 1981;141:891.
81. Ives HE, Daniel TO. Vascular Diseases of the Kidney. In BM Brenner, FC Rector (eds), The Kidney. Philadelphia: Saunders, 1991;1528.
82. Alpert BS, Bain HH, Balfe JW, et al. Role of the renin-angiotensin–aldosterone system in hypertensive children with coarctation of the aorta. Am J Cardiol 1979;43:828.
83. Simsolo R, Grunfeld B, Gimenez M, et al. Long-term systemic hypertension in children after successful repair of coarctation of the aorta. Am Heart J 1988;115:1268.
84. Mininberg DT, Roze S, Yoon HJ, Pearl M. Hypertension associated with crossed renal ectopia in an infant. Pediatrics 1971;48:454.
85. Loughbridge LW. Renal abnormalities in the Marfan syndrome. Q J Med 1959;28:531.
86. Neugarten J, Baldwin DS. Glomerulonephritis in bacterial endocarditis. Am J Med 1984;77:297.
87. Braunwald E. Valvular Heart Disease. In E Braunwald (ed), Heart Disease. A Textbook of Cardiovascular Medicine. Philadelphia: Saunders, 1988;1060.
88. Luscher TF, Lie JT, Stanson AW, et al. Arterial fibromuscular dysplasia. Mayo Clin Proc 1987;62:931.
89. Tilford DL, Kelsch RC. Renal artery stenosis in childhood neurofibromatosis. Am J Dis Child 1973;126:665.

90. Daniels SR, Loggie JMH, Schwartz DC, et al. Systemic hypertension secondary to peripheral vascular anomalies in patients with Williams syndrome. J Pediatr 1985;106:249.

91. Wiggelinkhuizen J, Cremin BJ. Takayasu arteritis and renovascular hypertension in childhood. Pediatrics 1978;62:209.

92. Daniels SR, Loggie JMH, McEnery PT, Towbin RB. Clinical spectrum of intrinsic renovascular hypertension in childhood. Pediatrics 1987;80:698.

93. Watson AR, Balfe JW, Hardy BE. Renovascular hypertension in childhood: a changing perspective in management. J Pediatr 1985;106:366.

94. Rahill WJ, Molteni A, Hawkins KM, et al. Hypertension and narrowing of the renal arteries in infancy. J Pediatr 1974;84:39.

95. Milner LS, Heitner R, Thomson PD, et al. Hypertension as the major problem of idiopathic arterial calcification of infancy. J Pediatr 1984;105:934.

96. McAlhany JC, Black HC, Hanback LD, Yarbrough DR. Renal arteriovenous fistula as a cause of hypertension. Am J Surg 1971;122:117.

97. Ullian ME, Molitoris BA. Bilateral congenital renal arteriovenous fistulas. Clin Nephrol 1987;27:293.

98. Klein I, Levey GS. New perspectives on thyroid hormone, catecholamines, and the heart. Am J Med 1984;76:167.

99. Resnick LM, Laragh JH. Plasma renin activity in syndromes of thyroid hormone excess and deficiency. Life Sci 1982;30:585.

100. Oberfield SE, Levine LS, New MI. Childhood hypertension due to adrenocorticoid disorders. Pediatr Ann 1982;11:623.

101. DiMartino-Nardi J, New MI. Low-renin hypertension of childhood. Pediatr Nephrol 1987;1:99.

102. Melby JC. Primary aldosteronism. Kidney Int 1984;26:769.

103. Farese RV, Biglieri EG, Shackleton CHL, et al. Licorice-induced hypermineralocorticoidism. N Engl J Med 1991;325:1223.

104. DeSanto NG, Giovambattista C, Giordano DR, Massimo L. Secondary forms of hypertension. Semin Nephrol 1989;9:272.

105. Lifton RP, Dluhy RG, Powers M, et al. Hereditary hypertension caused by chimaeric gene duplications and ectopic expression of aldosterone synthase. Nat Genet 1992;2:66.

106. Ganguly A, Gribble J, Tune B, et al. Renin-secreting Wilm's tumor with severe hypertension. Report of a case and brief review of renin-secreting tumors. Ann Intern Med 1973;79:835.

107. Mitchell JD, Baxter TJ, Blair-West JR, McCredie DA. Renin levels in nephroblastoma (Wilms' tumour). Report of a renin secreting tumour. Arch Dis Child 1970;45:376.

108. Corvol P, Pinet F, Galen FX, et al. Seven lessons from seven renin secreting tumors. Kidney Int 1988;34:38.

109. Warshaw BL, Anand SK, Olson DL, et al. Hypertension secondary to a renin-producing juxtaglomerular cell tumor. J Pediatr 1979;94:247.

110. Hinrose M, Arakawa K, Kikuchi M, et al. Primary reninism with renal hamartomatous alteration. JAMA 1974;230:1288.

111. Benowitz NL. Diagnosis and management of pheochromocytoma. Hosp Pract (Off Ed) 1990;25:95.

112. Bravo EL. Pheochromocytoma: new concepts and future trends. Kidney Int 1991;40:544.

113. Ein SH, Shandling B, Wesson D, Filler RM. Recurrent pheochromocytomas in children. J Pediatr Surg 1990;25:1063.
114. Bryer-Ash M, Wilson DM, Tune BM, et al. Hypertension caused by an aldosterone-secreting adenoma. Occurence in a 7-year-old child. Am J Dis Child 1984;138:673.
115. Weinblatt ME, Heisel MA, Siegel SE. Hypertension in children with neurologic tumors. Pediatrics 1983;71:947.
116. Saruta T, Saade GA, Kaplan NM. A possible mechanism for hypertension induced by oral contraceptives. Diminished feedback suppression of renin release. Arch Intern Med 1970;126:621.
117. Woods JW. Oral contraceptives and hypertension. Lancet 1967;2:653.
118. Riikonen R, Simell O, Dunkel L, et al. Hormonal background of the hypertension and fluid derangements associated with adrenocorticotrophic hormone treatment of infants. Eur J Pediatr 1989;148:737.
119. Roche H, Hyman G, Nahas G. Hypertension and intravenous antidopaminergic drugs. N Engl J Med 1985;312:1125.
120. Sheridan C, Chandra P, Jacinto M, Greenwald ES. Transient hypertension after high doses of metoclopramide. N Engl J Med 1982;307:1346.
121. Vogelzang NJ. Hypertension after metoclopramide. N Engl J Med 1983;308:780.
122. Saken R, Kates GL, Miller K. Drug-induced hypertension in infancy. J Pediatr 1979;95:1077.
123. Metz S, Klein C, Morton N. Rebound hypertension after discontinuation of transdermal clonidine therapy. Am J Med 1987;82:17.
124. Kahan BD. Cyclosporine. N Engl J Med 1989;321:1725.
125. Kletzel M, Jaffe N. Systemic hypertension: a complication of intra-arterial cis-diammine dichloroplatinum (II) infusion. Cancer 1981;47:245.
126. Offner G, Hoyer PF, Latta K, et al. One year's experience with recombinant erythropoietin in children undergoing continuous ambulatory or cycling peritoneal dialysis. Pediatr Nephrol 1990;4:498.
127. Erslev AJ. Erythropoietin. N Engl J Med 1991;324:1339.
128. Ritz E, Mann J, Stoeppler M. Lead and the kidney. In J-P Grünfeld, JF Bach, J Crosnier, et al (eds), Advances in Nephrology. Chicago: Year Book, 1988;17:241.
129. Foulds DM, Copeland KC, Franks RC. Mercury poisoning and acrodynia. Am J Dis Child 1987;141:124.
130. Sofer S, Gueron M. Vasodilators and hypertensive encephalopathy following scorpian envenomation in children. Chest 1990;97:118.
131. Baer L, Radichevich I. Cigarette smoking in hypertensive patients. Blood pressure and endocrine responses. Am J Med 1985;78:564.
132. Robertson D, Hollister AS, Kincaid D, et al. Caffeine and hypertension. Am J Med 1984;77:54.
133. Robertson CS, Clifton GL, Taylor AA, Grossman RG. Treatment of hypertension associated with head injury. J Neurosurg 1983;59:455.
134. Wallace JD, Levy LL. Blood pressure after stroke. JAMA 1981;246:2177.
135. Lichtenfeld P. Autonomic dysfunction in the Guillain-Barré syndrome. Am J Med 1971;50:772.
136. Pelligra SJ. Severe hypertension due to autonomic dysreflexia. JAMA 1986;256:1137.

137. Guyton AC. The Kidney in Blood Pressure Control and Hypertension. In MA Holliday, TM Barratt, RL Vernier (eds), Pediatric Nephrology. Baltimore: Williams & Wilkins, 1987:729.
138. Marquez JM, Douglas ME, Downs JB, et al. Renal function and cardiovascular responses during positive airway pressure. Anesthesiology 1979;50:393.
139. Ross RD, Daniels SR, Loggie JMH, et al. Sleep apnea–associated hypertension and reversible left ventricular hypertrophy. J Pediatr 1987;111:253.
140. Hamdan JA, Taleb YA, Ahmed MS. Traction-induced hypertension in children. Clin Orthop 1984;185:87.
141. Turner MC, Ruley EJ, Buckley KM, Strife CF. Blood pressure elevation in children with orthopedic immobilization. J Pediatr 1979;95:989.
142. Linshaw MA, Stapleton FB, Gruskin AB, et al. Traction-related hypertension in children. J Pediatr 1979;95:994.
143. Redman CWG. Hypertension in pregnancy: a case discussion. Kidney Int 1987;32:151.
144. Cunningham FG, Lindheimer MD. Hypertension in pregnancy. N Engl J Med 1992;326:927.
145. Ruddel H, Langewitz W, Schachinger H, et al. Hemodynamic response patterns to mental stress: diagnostic and therapeutic implications. Am Heart J 1988;116:617.
146. Noble-Jamieson G, Barnes ND, Thiru S, Mowat AP. Severe hypertension after liver transplantation in alpha 1 antitrypsin deficiency. Arch Dis Child 1990;65:1217.
147. Gruskin AB, Fleischmann L. Clinical quiz. Pediatr Nephrol 1990;4:578.

CHAPTER 4

Diagnostic Evaluation of Hypertension in Children

Marva M. Moxey-Mims

The prevalence of childhood hypertension is reported to be 1–5% [1, 2]. Unfortunately, there are no data in the pediatric literature on the prospective outcome of mildly hypertensive, asymptomatic children with regard to long-term morbidity. However, the awareness of the cardiovascular risks of prolonged hypertension in adults, combined with the belief that adult hypertension likely originates in childhood, has led to the more routine measurement of blood pressure (BP) in children. It is generally thought that early detection and proper evaluation of this disorder in children, combined with appropriate early intervention, can lead to a decrease in the risks for morbidity and mortality. The majority of hypertensive children have mild elevations in BP, and the diagnosis of primary, or essential, hypertension predominates even in very young children [3]. However, approximately 10% of hypertensive children have very high BP. The majority of these children are found to have secondary hypertension. The challenge facing the physicians who care for these children is minimizing the potential of missing the diagnosis of a "curable" form of hypertension without subjecting every child to the risks (and expense) of invasive tests and protracted laboratory investigations.

It is generally assumed that the younger the child, the higher the BP, or the greater the number of known risk factors for organic disease, the more aggressive the work-up should be. In young children with a high risk factor for organic disease, a secondary, and potentially curable cause for hypertension is most likely to be found. By far, the greatest proportion of these secondary causes are either renal or renovascular in origin [4].

In children, hypertension is defined as average systolic or diastolic BP greater than or equal to the ninety-fifth percentile for age and sex on at least three occasions [5]. Most physicians are cognizant of the need for repeated measurements to establish the diagnosis of persistent hypertension, but in children, this must be coupled with a knowledge of the physiologic maturational differences in children of the same chronologic age [5–12]. Height appears to be the most sensitive indicator and has been shown to correlate with BP independent of chronologic age [6–10]. It is therefore recommended that "height-age" (the chronologic age for which height is at the fiftieth percentile on a standard growth chart) be used to verify the diagnosis of childhood hypertension [6, 7]. Weight also correlates with BP. However, the higher BP in an obese child is unlikely to be physiologic [5–7, 11, 13].

Borderline Hypertension

Borderline, or mildly elevated BP (see Chapter 2), should be measured repeatedly over several months. In cases of borderline hypertension, office BP measurements have been shown to be poor predictors of average 24-hour ambulatory BP [14]; this may be related to the "white coat" syndrome [15]. In these situations, ambulatory BP monitoring (ABPM) can be an indispensable tool (see Chapter 2). Several companies now market automatic and semiautomatic ambulatory BP monitors. The BP readings obtained in this manner have been shown to give a reliable assessment of the average BP level [16–20]. In addition, when compared with office measurements, ABPM measurements have been shown to more accurately predict the severity of end-organ damage [21–23]. These devices are now available with varying cuff sizes, making them suitable for use in pediatrics.

Moderate Hypertension

Before initiating specific evaluation, moderate to severe BP elevation deserves repeated checks over a shorter period of time than mild BP elevation. Office measurements in these instances have been shown to correlate with the average 24-hour ambulatory BP [14]. Indications for the use of a 24-hour ABPM include (1) office ausculatory or automated readings different from home ausculatory or electronic BP readings, (2) noncompliant patients, (3) adolescents with borderline BP, (4) variable readings in young children and adolescents, (5) assessment of the effect of mild to moderate activity on BP, and (6) patients on multiple antihypertensive drugs without normalization of BP. In some instances, 24-hour monitoring reveals an abnormal noctural BP pattern. Under normal circumstances, BP is lower during the night than the day. If the reverse is detected, it is suggestive of chronic renal failure, sleep apnea, pheochromocytoma, diabetes mellitus, Cushing's syndrome, or congestive heart failure.

Severe Hypertension

Severe, acute, usually transient hypertension can be seen in numerous situations in which treatment is required. No further evaluation of the hypertension is warranted unless the hypertension persists after resolution of the precipitating episode. Precipitating episodes include burns, fracture, orthopedic traction, abdominal pain, laceration, dental extraction, and the time during or immediately after anesthesia [2]. Usually BP returns to normal after resolution of the acute event. Undoubtedly, in all hypertensive emergencies (see Chapter 6), treatment takes precedence over evaluation.

Evaluating Hypertensive Children

Two of the most important goals in the evaluation of hypertension are to obtain a complete medical history and to determine whether the child is genuinely hypertensive. The historical information should include family history, neonatal history, dietary habits, review of systems, and ingestion of drugs (prescription, over-the-counter, or illicit) (Table 4.1). In infants and young children, a neonatal history is important because of the frequent use of umbilical artery catheters and the subsequent increase in the occurrence of renovascular hypertension in these children (see Chapter 3). A history of significant abdominal or back trauma may point to potential renal or renovascular etiologies. A history of drug use or abuse should also be sought (e.g., cold preparations [sympathomimetics], oral contraceptives, anabolic steroids, amphetamines, and cocaine) (Table 4.2). Patients and parents should also be questioned about potential toxic or chemical exposures (e.g., heavy metals [lead–either present exposure or past history of plumbism] or solvents). A detailed history of family members with hypertension is needed. The history should include the age of onset, any incidence of stroke or heart attack (along with age of occurrence), renal disease, collagen vascular disease, and mucocutaneous syndromes.

The review of systems may be valuable in revealing symptoms of possible associated diseases. Examples of such symptoms and their associated diseases include unexplained fevers (possible pyelonephritis or recurrent urinary tract infection [UTI]); leg pain with exercise (coarctation); polyuria, weakness, and muscle cramps (hyperaldosteronism); weight loss, fine tremor, and sweating (hyperthyroidism); and sweating and palpitations (pheochromocytoma).

A physical examination may point out possible secondary causes of hypertension, while also assessing clinical end-organ damage (Table 4.3). In this examination, BP should be measured in upper and lower extremities

TABLE 4.1
Historical Information Relevant to the Diagnosis of Hypertension

Information	Relevance
Family history of hypertension, pre-eclampsia, renal disease, tumors	Important in essential hypertension, inherited renal diseases, familial pheochromocytoma
Family history of early complications of hypertension and/or atherosclerosis	Suggests likely course of hypertension and/or presence of other coronary artery risk factors
Neonatal history	Use of umbilical artery catheter suggests need to evaluate renal vasculature and kidneys
Dietary history	Assessment of sodium and caloric intake
Headaches, dizziness, epistaxis, visual problems	Nonspecific symptomatology
Adbominal pain, dysuria, frequency, nocturia, enuresis	May suggest underlying renal pathology
Joint pains or swelling, or facial or peripheral edema	Suggestive of connective tissue disease and/or other forms of nephritis
Weight loss, failure to gain weight with good appetite, excess sweating, pallor, fevers, constipation	In combination suggest pheochromo- cytoma
Muscle cramps, weakness, constipation	May suggest hyperaldosteronism with hypokalemia
Age of onset of menarche	May be helpful in suggesting hydroxy- lase deficiencies
Ingestion of prescription and over-the- counter drugs, contraceptives, illicit drugs	Drug-induced hypertension

Source: Modified from JMH Loggie. Evaluation of the Hypertensive Child and Adolescent. In JMH Loggie (ed), Pediatric and Adolescent Hypertension. Boston: Blackwell, 1992;112.

to rule out coarctation of the aorta. A high pulse rate may be indicative of hyperdynamic states (e.g., hyperthyroidism). Height and weight should be checked to rule out growth retardation (which is often seen in chronic renal disease), many endocrine disorders, or other chronic illnesses. The skin should be carefully examined: Striae, acne, and hirsutism can be seen in Cushing's disease or anabolic steroid use; café-au-lait spots may indicate the possibility of neurofibromatosis; and adenoma sebaceum may suggest the possibility of tuberous sclerosis. Ambiguous genitalia/virilization make adrenal hyperplasia a possibility. Joint pains or rash may raise suspicion for systemic lupus erythematosus. Girls should be examined for the stigmata of Turner's syndrome, such as webbed neck and shield chest. The abdominal examination for both girls and boys should include not only

TABLE 4.2
Some Prescription and Nonprescription Drugs That May Cause Hypertension*

Albuterol
Amphetamines (biphetamine, dexedrine)
Amphotericin B
Antidepressants (amitriptyline, imipramine, Ativan)
Antipsychotics (Haldol)
Bromocriptine
Caffeine
Calderol
Carbamazepine (Tegretol)
Cocaine
Cyclosporine
Dexadrine
Dihydroergotamine
Dimercaprol
Ephedrine
Epinephrine
Epogen
Ethanol
Fentanyl
Gentamicin
Ketoconazole
Metaproterenol
Methylphenidate (Ritalin)
Metoclopramide HCl (Reglan)
Naphazoline HCl
Nonsteroidal anti-inflammatory drugs (ibuprofen, naproxen)
Oral contraceptives
Oxymetazoline HCl
Phenylephrine HCl
Phenylpropanolamine HCl
Promethazine HCl (Phenergan)
Pseudoephedrine HCl
Steroids (hydrocortisone, Medrol, prednisone)
Terbutaline
Tetrahydrozoline HCl
Vincristine
Xylometazoline HCl

*Some of the drugs listed are ingredients in many over-the-counter medications. Please refer to the package label. In addition, please refer to the Physicians Desk Reference or package inserts for potential interaction with other drugs.

TABLE 4.3
Findings on Physical Examination Useful in the Evaluation of Childhood
Hypertension

	Finding	*Potential Hypertensive Etiology*
Vital signs	Tachycardia	Anemia
		Hyperthyroidism
		Pheochromocytoma
	Postural hypotension	Pheochromocytoma
	Decreased/delayed femoral pulses	Coarctation of aorta
	Differential blood pressures (upper extremities > lower)	Coarctation of aorta
Height/weight	Growth retardation	Chronic renal disease
		Cushing's syndrome
	Truncal obesity	Cushing's syndrome
Head, eyes, ear, nose, and throat	Moon facies	Cushing's syndrome
	Elfin facies	Williams syndrome
	Webbed neck	Turner's syndrome
	Thyromegaly	Hyperthyroidism
	Buffalo hump	Cushing's syndrome
Skin	Pallor, flushing, increased perspiration	Pheochromocytoma
		Hyperdynamic essential hypertension
	Acne, hirsutism, striae	Cushing's syndrome
		Anabolic steroid use
	Café-au-lait spots, neurofibromas	Neurofibromatosis
	Adenoma sebaceum	Tuberous sclerosis
	Butterfly rash	Systemic lupus erythematosus
Chest	Wide-spaced nipples/shield chest	Turner's syndrome
	Heart murmur	Coarctation of aorta
		Anemia
Abdomen	Palpable mass	Wilms' tumor
		Neuroblastoma
		Pheochromocytoma
		Polycystic kidneys
		Hydronephrosis
		Trauma
	Epigastric or flank bruit	Coarctation of aorta
		Renal artery stenosis
		Trauma
		Arteritis
	Mass	Wilms' tumor
		Polycystic kidney disease
		Neuroblastoma
Genitalia	Ambiguous/virilization	Adrenal hyperplasia

Extremities	Joint swelling or tenderness	Systemic lupus erythematosus
	Muscle weakness	Hyperaldosteronism
	Edema	Renal disease
	Tetany	Hyperaldosteronism
Neurologic	Bell's palsy	Chronic hypertension

TABLE 4.4
Basic Laboratory Tests for Initial Childhood Hypertensive Evaluation

Complete blood count
Urinalysis
Urine culture
BUN, creatinine
Plasma renin activity
Uric acid
Electrolytes and total CO_2
Cholesterol and triglycerides
Echocardiogram

palpation for masses but also a careful auscultation for bruits to rule out arteriovenous malformations or stenoses. Funduscopic examination is often not helpful, especially in younger children, even when severe hypertension is present. However, changes such as hemorrhages, exudates, and papilledema may be present in adolescents. Many times only mild changes such as arteriolar narrowing or spasm and arteriovenous thickening are seen with funduscopic examination. Bell's palsy, a significant neurologic finding, has been noted as the presenting sign in some cases of childhood hypertension [24, 25].

Basic laboratory tests in any child with hypertension should include a complete blood cell count (CBC), urinalysis, urine culture, blood urea nitrogen (BUN), creatinine, plasma renin activity, uric acid, electrolytes, cholesterol and triglycerides (fasting), and echocardiogram (Table 4.4 and Figure 4.1). These tests give insight into the potential etiology of the hypertension, as well as evaluating potential atherosclerosis risk factors and the existence of end-organ damage. A normal CBC readily rules out both polycythemia and anemia as the causes of hypertension. Likewise, a normal urinalysis usually rules out acute glomerulonephritis. Although electrolytes are usually normal, abnormalities may result from adrenal impairment (hypokalemia, hypernatremia, or alkalosis) or underlying renal disease (hyperkalemia or metabolic acidosis). Uric acid is often elevated in people with early essential hypertension without clinical evidence of impaired renal function [26, 27], as well as those with

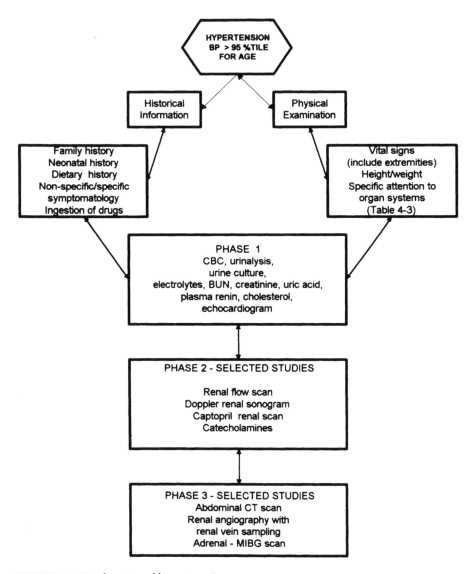

FIGURE 4.1. Evaluation of hypertension.

hypertension secondary to structural renal disease. An M-mode echocardiogram is the best test to assess left ventricular wall mass and chamber size, as well as left atrial chamber size, as an indicator of the chronicity of hypertension.

In severely hypertensive patients, peripheral plasma renin activity (PRA) is a useful screen for hypertension secondary to stimulation of the renin-angiotensin–aldosterone system or mineralocorticoid excess. It is

TABLE 4.5
Normal Values for Pediatric Plasma Renin Activity (PRA)

Age	Mean PRA in ng/ml/hr (range)
3 days–3 mos	12.0 (0.5–24.2)
3–12 mos	5.7 (2.2–10.2)
1–3 yrs	3.1 (0.5–8.0)
3–6 yrs	2.8 (0.1–12.0)
6–9 yrs	2.0 (0.1–7.5)
9–12 yrs	2.0 (0.2–7.0)
12–15 yrs	1.9 (0.2–8.0)
15–18 yrs	1.5 (0.2–6.5)

Source: Summarized from LB Hiner, AB Gruskin, HJ Baluarte, et al. Plasma renin activity in normal children. J Pediatr 1976;89:258; HP Stalker, NH Holland, JM Kotchen, et al. Plasma renin activity in healthy children. J Pediatr 1976;89:256; and TJW Fiselier, P Lijnen, L Monnens, et al. Levels of renin, angiotensin I and II, angiotensin-converting enzyme, and aldosterone in infancy and childhood. Eur J Pediatr 1983;141:3.

expected to be elevated in the former, low in the latter. However, it must be remembered that PRA values are normally higher in infants and children [28–31] and even in adolescents [32] when compared with adults (Table 4.5). One must also keep in mind that PRA increases when plasma volume is decreased, salt intake is restricted, or the patient is in an upright position. Despite the known inverse relationship of sodium excretion (as a reflection of sodium intake) to PRA, Hiner and colleagues showed that this relationship did not persist when the rate of sodium excretion was corrected for body surface area [28]. In addition, children on an unrestricted diet are unlikely to have a sodium excretion rate low enough (<50 mEq/24 hours) to account for an abnormally elevated PRA [30]. Profiling of sodium excretion rates is therefore unnecessary unless there is particular cause for concern about an unusual diet. It is important to note, however, that many medications, especially antihypertensives, can increase or decrease PRA (Table 4.6).

Children with Possible Secondary Hypertension

As previously stated, the majority of children with elevated BPs have essential hypertension. However, for the small group with secondary hypertension, specific disease cure rates are reported at 70–90%, especially when the etiology is unilateral renovascular disease [34–36]. It is therefore important to identify this group since without a cure, antihypertensive medications are a lifelong commitment, and we do not know the consequences of such prolonged treatment initiated in childhood.

TABLE 4.6
Medications Affecting Plasma Renin Activity (PRA)*

Medication	Effect on PRA
Diuretics	↑
Hydralazine	↑
Diazoxide	↑
Nitroprusside	↑
Minoxidil	↑
ACE inhibitors	↑
Aldomet	↓
Beta blockers	↓
Clonidine	↓
Calcium channel blockers*	↔
Oral contraceptives	↑
Gentamicin	↑

↑= increase; ↓ = decrease; ↔ = no effect.
*The exception is short-acting nifedipine, which causes a short-term increase in PRA with return to normal levels 4 hours after the dose [33].
Source: JH Bauer, S Sunderrajan, G Reams. Effects of calcium entry blockers on renin–angiotensin–aldosterone system, renal function and hemodynamics, salt and water excretion and body fluid composition. Am J Cardiol 1985;56:62.

Renovascular Hypertension

The exact prevalence of renovascular hypertension is unknown. Children with renovascular hypertension usually have moderate to severe BP elevations, many of them asymptomatic. In some instances, however, these children may present acutely with encephalopathy or stroke. Growth failure may be seen in some, though most are of normal height and weight. While it is important to listen for abdominal bruits in children suspected of having renovascular disease, the absence of this finding does not rule out this possibility. The auscultation should be particularly concentrated over the epigastric and flank areas. The occurrence of bruits in children with proven renal artery disease has been reported to range from 37% to 57% [2, 37]. Although the average age of presentation of renovascular hypertension is 9–10 years [38], increasing numbers of infants with a past history of indwelling umbilical artery catheters are being found to have renovascular hypertension [39]. Interestingly, it seems that in the absence of neurofibromatosis, black children rarely manifest this disorder [2].

In most children with renovascular hypertension, the history, physical, and basic laboratory tests are not very informative. The peripheral PRA may be high, but this is not diagnostic, and in some instances it may actually be normal. Therefore, more specific diagnostic studies must be undertaken in children for whom there is a high index of suspicion (Figure 4.2). Attempts

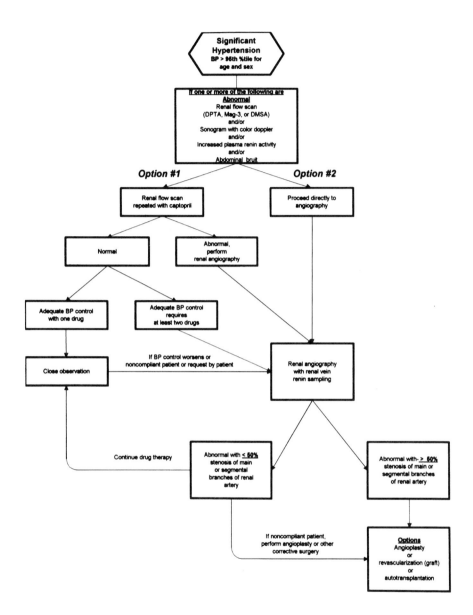

FIGURE 4.2. Evaluation of renovascular hypertension.

have been made to evaluate the effect of captopril administration on PRA levels, the theory being that the PRA should increase more in patients with renovascular lesions than those without. Results have been mixed in adults, with good differentiation reported by some [40] and lower sensitivities reported by others [41, 42]. The results have also been mixed in children. One group

TABLE 4.7
Radiologic Tests Used in the Assessment of Renovascular Hypertension

Test	Abnormal Findings
Excretory urogram	Hyperconcentration of contrast
	Delayed excretion of contrast
	Discrepancy in kidney size
	Ureteral or pelvic notching
Radionuclide imaging	
^{99}Tc-DTPA	Delayed/asymmetric transit of radiopharma-
	ceutical
^{99}Tc-DMSA	Focal abnormalities
	Asymmetric renal size
	Asymmetric distribution of radiopharmaceutical
Ultrasound	Kidney size discrepancies
	Thrombi
	Vascular luminal narrowing
	Increased echogenicity
Digital subtraction angiography	Visualization of abdominal aorta and renal
	arteries
Conventional angiography	Visualization of abdominal aorta and renal
	arteries

reported a greater PRA response to captopril in children with renovascular disease than those without, although actual numbers were not given [43]. They did find a significant correlation between the BP response to a dose of captopril and the patient's initial PRA, making this a potentially useful screening test for high-renin hypertension in situations in which it may not be easy to obtain a PRA. Patients whose systolic BP decreased by a mean of 10% or whose diastolic BP decreased by 15% were found to have an elevated PRA. A more recent, though smaller, study found only a 43% positive predictive value for the captopril stimulation of PRA [44]. Both studies used a dose of 0.7 mg/kg of captopril and measured BP and PRA before and after the dose. The post-dose measurements were performed at 1 [44] or 2 hours [43] after the captopril administration. This test will require further evaluation to determine its usefulness and to establish the optimal time to check for a response.

Diagnostic Tests for Renovascular Hypertension

The definitive diagnostic study for renovascular hypertension is the arteriogram (discussed below). However, because of the highly invasive nature of this test and the risk of complications, it should be reserved for children in whom the probability of demonstrating an abnormality is highest. There are, therefore, numerous screening tests used to narrow the field so that every child need not undergo arteriography (Table 4.7).

Excretory Urography (Intravenous Pyelogram). The excretory urogram has traditionally been used as a screening test for renovascular hypertension. Positive findings in unilateral renal artery stenosis include hyperconcentration of contrast material, delayed excretion of contrast, discrepancy in kidney sizes (ischemic kidney is shorter), and ureteral or pelvic notching (which are considered to be evidence of collateral circulation) [45] (Figure 4.3).The most common abnormality is the discrepancy in renal length, which is defined arbitrarily as greater than or equal to 0.5 cm difference between the two kidneys in children less than 15 years old, and greater than or equal to 1.0 cm difference in those over 15 years of age [37]. The other radiologic findings are rarely seen in children. The reported percentage of abnormal excretory urograms in children ranges from 32% to 65% in unilateral disease, and from 20% to 50% in bilateral disease [36, 46]. This compares with rates of 80% and 60% in adults for unilateral and bilateral disease, respectively [39, 47]. The lower sensitivity in pediatrics is presumably related to the higher prevalence of bilateral and intrarenal arterial lesions. This test is not generally considered to be a reliable screen in pediatrics, but it is still used in some centers because of the ease of performance and ready availability. Although it can be useful in detecting other renal abnormalities such as cortical scarring, obstructive uropathy, renal masses (cysts, tumors), or atrophy resulting from chronic diffuse parenchymal disease, many would argue that for these abnormalities, ultrasonography would be equally informative if not superior (see below).

Radionuclide Imaging. Radionuclide imaging is particularly useful in the neonatal period when renal functional immaturity results in poor excretion of contrast material and inadequate visualization of the kidneys by excretory urography. The advantage in all age groups is the ability to quantitate both total and individual renal function and the lack of adverse reactions. The disadvantage is poor anatomic resolution when compared with other imaging methods.

Several different types of radiopharmaceuticals exist, but there are currently two that are generally applied to the assessment of suspected renovascular hypertension. The first is ^{99m}Tc-diethylenetriamine-pentaacetic acid (DTPA). This agent is excreted by glomerular filtration and provides a measure of glomerular filtration rate (GFR). Because its distribution is proportional to renal blood flow and glomerular filtration, relative individual renal function can be quantitated by determination of radionuclide activity in the kidney during the first 1–3 minutes after injection of DTPA. This particular agent has been reported to have a sensitivity of 82–91% with a specificity of 90% for the diagnosis of renovascular hypertension in adults [48, 49]. An abnormal finding is generally defined as one in which there is delayed or asymmetric transit of the radiopharmaceutical due to obstruction of the affected artery (Figure 4.4). However, a study of pediatric patients showed this test to have a sensitivity of only 54% for the detec-

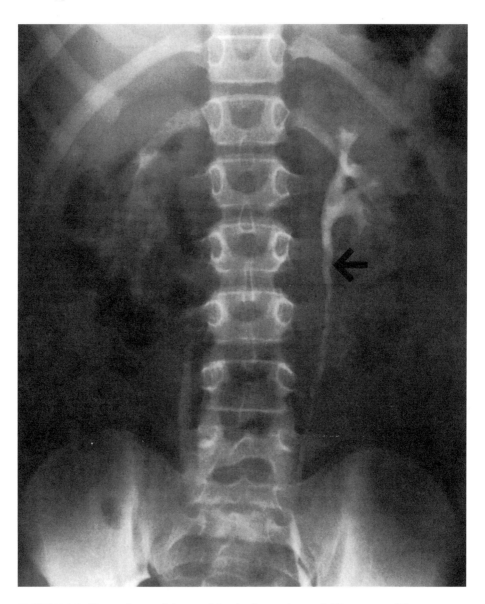

FIGURE 4.3. Ureteral or pelvic notching is shown (arrow). (Courtesy of Department of Radiology, Children's Hospital of Buffalo.)

tion of renovascular hypertension [50]. Administration of captopril has been reported to increase the sensitivity of this test, often after a single dose [51–54]. This enhancement of ^{99m}Tc-DTPA scintigraphic abnormalities occurs because the angiotensin II–dependent GFR in renal artery stenosis is short-circuited by captopril, preventing the formation of

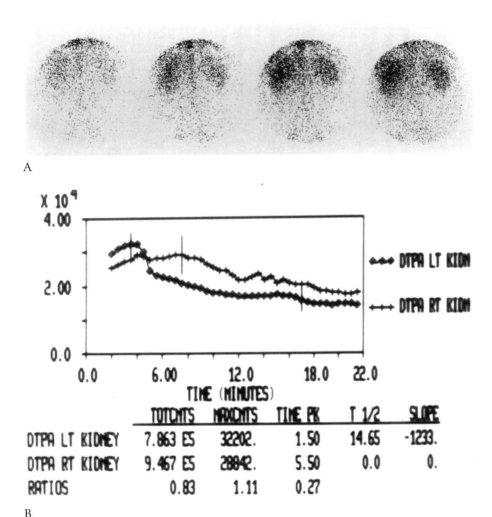

FIGURE 4.4. A. There is delayed or asymmetric transit of the radiopharmaceutical due to obstruction of the affected artery. The appearance of the kidneys is delayed. B. The curve for the right kidney demonstrates a lower and delayed peak. (Courtesy of Department of Radiology, Children's Hospital of Buffalo.)

angiotensin II. The resultant decrease in GFR is reflected in a decreased renal excretion of DTPA. The specificity of this test in adults varies from 73% to 100%, and the sensitivity varies from 48% to 100%, both depending on the characteristics of the population studied. A report including children described a dramatic but reversible deterioration of function in the affected kidney detected with ^{99m}Tc-DTPA scintigraphy [55]. In kidneys without a stenotic artery no deterioration in function was seen. There are no controlled, prospective studies of this phenomenon reported in the pediatric literature.

The second type of radiopharmeceutical used for radionuclide imaging is Tc-dimercaptosuccinate (DMSA), which is extracted by the renal tubules. Approximately 40% of DMSA is retained in the renal cortex for prolonged periods. Delayed imaging provides a sensitive means to detect focal renal cortical lesions that may be missed by excretory urography. It can also be used to detect regional and differential renal function [56], although this may be unreliable in cases of urinary tract obstruction if a significant quantity of isotope is retained in the collecting system. This radionuclide has been reported by some to be more sensitive than ^{99m}Tc-DTPA in screening for renovascular or renal parenchymal hypertension [50, 57]. Rosen reported a sensitivity of 92% for this test, as compared with sensitivities of 54% and 60% for ^{99m}Tc-DTPA and excretory urography, respectively. An abnormal ^{99m}Tc-DMSA scan was defined as revealing focal abnormalities (Figure 4.5), asymmetric renal size, or asymmetric distribution of the radioactive tracer [50]. Because of the significant improvement in sensitivity over ^{99m}Tc-DTPA and excretory urography, this study is certainly worth considering early in the evaluation of the patient with possible renovascular hypertension.

Ultrasound.   Ultrasound is particularly useful in neonates, in whom hypertension is most frequently related to thrombosis after umbilical artery catheterization. The aorta, inferior vena cava, and their major branches are usually well delineated in neonates with an arterial thrombus showing up as an abnormal echogenic focus in the vessel lumen (Figure 4.6). The focus is often associated with luminal narrowing [58]. The ultrasound findings in venous thrombosis vary with the stage of disease [59]. In the acute stage of the disease, there is renal enlargement and decreased cortical echogenicity. Later, the kidney appears echogenic and severe atrophy results if there is no collateral formation or recanalization. If there is no collateral formation or recanalization, there is increased parenchymal echogenicity, loss of corticomedullary definition, and often calcifications. The thrombus itself may be visualized in the renal vein or inferior vena cava.

During and after the neonatal period, ultrasound is also useful for assessing abdominal masses that may be impinging on renal vasculature, determining renal size, and demonstrating renal scarring. The ultrasound cannot, however, indicate renal function and may miss some areas of scarring, especially in the upper renal poles where rib acoustic shadows may interfere with the image. These shortcomings can be compensated for by using ultrasound in conjunction with radionuclide imaging. Because ultrasonography is operator-dependent, the physician evaluating the hypertensive patient needs to know the level of expertise and competence of the operator when deciding whether to use this modality to evaluate a hypertensive patient.

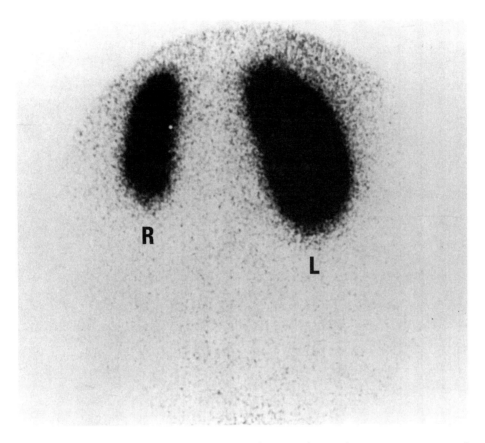

FIGURE 4.5. The right kidney (R) is somewhat atrophic with a DMSA trapping of only 25% of the total. (Courtesy of Department of Radiology, Children's Hospital of Buffalo.)

Digital Subtraction Angiography. Digital subtraction angiography (DSA) can be performed intravenously (IVDSA) or intra-arterially (IADSA). IVDSA allows visualization of the arterial system after injection of contrast material. A computer subtracts the venous images, leaving the abdominal aorta and renal arteries clearly visible (Figure 4.7). It has been used in adults since the early 1980s and is accepted in this population as a suitable procedure for the initial evaluation of patients with suspected renovascular hypertension [60, 61]. A review of the adult literature shows a sensitivity of 87.6%, with a specificity of 89.5% for demonstrating arterial lesions [62]. It was noted, however, that approximately 7.4% of the time this study can be nondiagnostic, resulting in an overall predictive value comparable to that of the excretory urogram.

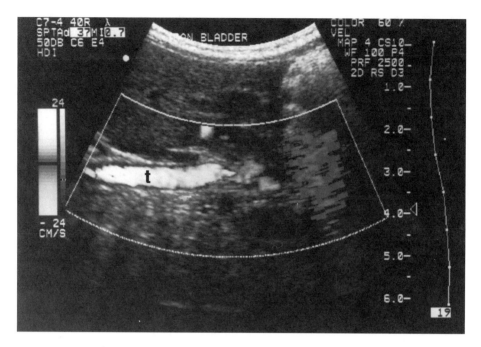

FIGURE 4.6. The aorta contains a significant-sized thrombus (t). (Courtesy of Department of Radiology, Children's Hospital of Buffalo.)

The only published reports of IVDSA studies in children found that all major vessels arising from the aorta and their branches were easily seen [63]. The intrarenal vessels were seen in some cases, but intrarenal veins were never visible. No renal vessel abnormalities were encountered, so a detection rate could not be determined.

The major advantage of IVDSA is that it only requires venous catheterization, usually of the superior vena cava (SVC). However, this can be a disadvantage in pediatrics, because it is often difficult to catheterize the SVC in small children. This procedure has also been performed via peripheral veins, but only in adults [64]. Other problems include a lack of patient cooperation in the pediatric age group, intestinal peristalsis, and increased amounts of bowel gas, all of which can degrade the image [65]. Additionally, the examination is nonselective, so smaller intrarenal vessels are poorly seen and it may be difficult to distinguish renal vessels from overlying mesenterics. The inability to see intrarenal vessels clearly is particularly relevant in pediatrics because a large proportion of stenoses in children are located in segmental or more distal arterial branches. Additionally, because IVDSA requires 50% more iodine, the risk of contrast-induced complications is even higher than with an excretory urogram.

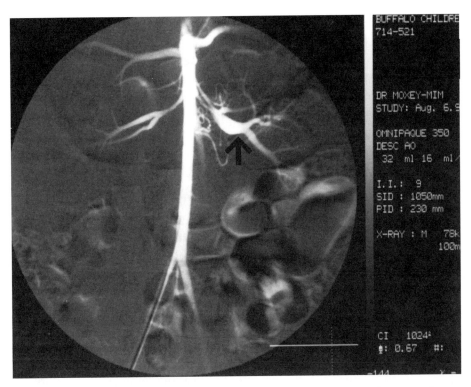

FIGURE 4.7. Digital subtraction angiography permits computer analysis to subtract venous images, leaving the abdominal aorta and renal arteries clearly visible. The arrow shows the poststenotic dilatation. (Courtesy of Department of Radiology, Children's Hospital of Buffalo.)

Overall, the role of IVDSA in young children is unclear. Technical issues are less of a problem in older children and adolescents; therefore it may be a useful study in these groups.

IADSA is no less invasive than conventional arteriography. However, smaller volumes of contrast are required because of the better contrast resolution of digital imaging. Therefore, the risk of contrast-induced complications is reduced. It is thought that IADSA is a potentially superior method for diagnosing intrarenal vascular pathology, including distal branch lesions [66]. As with IVDSA, experience in children is limited.

Arteriography.   Arteriography is still the definitive method for the diagnosis of renovascular abnormalities in children. The study is less risky if performed after the BP is under some degree of medical control. Arteriography is indicated in those with severe hypertension and those in whom screening studies strongly suggest renovascular hypertension.

A complete study includes injections of both renal arteries to determine whether or not there are bilateral lesions. In children, the renal arteries are approached by percutaneous puncture of a femoral artery with retrograde catheterization of the abdominal aorta. The radiographic findings in renal artery stenosis depend on its etiology. Medial fibromuscular dysplasia is the most common pathology of renal artery stenosis in childhood. The peripheral vessels are involved as often as the main artery, and there is often bilateral disease. The "chain of beads" appearance described in adults is reported in only 10% of pediatric patients [36]. This disease is not necessarily limited to the renal vessels but may be seen in a generalized distribution in some patients, including the carotid, vertebral, and mesenteric arteries, as well as the aorta.

Neurofibromatosis is the second most common cause of renovascular disease in children [36, 67]. Findings include renal artery stenosis, often associated with aneurysms [68, 69]. The stenoses are usually found at or near the origin of the main renal arteries.

The mere finding of a stenotic lesion, however, does not mean that it is the source of the patient's hypertension. It is unusual for stenoses of the renal artery to produce hypertension unless the vessel is narrowed by more than 50%. During arteriography, evidence of collateral circulation should also be sought, as this usually implies that the stenotic lesion is hemodynamically significant (Figure 4.8). In studies, the presence of collaterals positively correlates with a successful surgical outcome [46, 70]. Hemodynamically insignificant stenoses have been found in both hypertensive and normotensive people [71, 72].

The primary means of determining the functional significance of a renal artery stenosis has been, and still is, to measure renal vein renins. These measurements can be used in calculations in the following ways:

1.   A ratio of renal venous renins from one kidney to the other of 1.5 to 1.0 or greater (termed *lateralizing*) has been used to predict potential cure of hypertension by correction of the lesion [73]. This ratio is helpful, but in and of itself, is not 100% predictive. There have been patients, particularly those with severe bilateral lesions or with segmental lesions, who have been surgically cured despite having ratios of less than 1.5 [74]. Numerous attempts have been made to capitalize on the effect that many antihypertensive medications have on PRA (see Table 4.6), in order to "stimulate" or "unmask" a lateralizing renal venous renin ratio. Drugs used have included intravenous hydralazine [75–78], continuous sodium nitroprusside intravenous infusion [79], intravenous diazoxide [80], and more recently oral captopril at various dosages [81–83]. The best results have been documented after hydralazine and captopril stimulation. These studies have reported improvements in the rate of lateralization in patients with unilateral disease from 60–80% to 80–100%, before and after stimulation, respectively. In patients with bilateral disease, lateral-

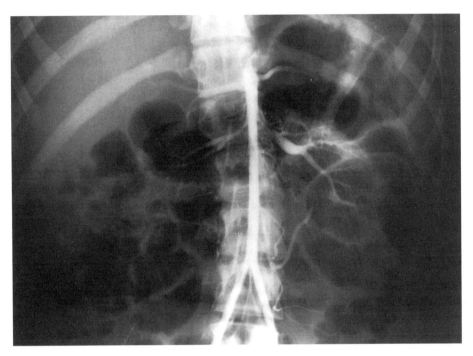

FIGURE 4.8. Conventional arteriography demonstrating evidence of collateral circulation implicating that a stenotic lesion is hemodynamically significant. (Courtesy of Department of Radiology, Children's Hospital of Buffalo.)

ization rates have increased from 20–60% before stimulation to 40–100% after stimulation. There are no significant changes in the renal venous renin ratios in patients with hemodynamically insignificant lesions or essential hypertension [77, 83]. Because of the risk for nonoliguric reversible renal failure associated with captopril, it would not be prudent to carry out such a stimulation test with hydralazine or a single dose of captopril in patients with either a stenosis to a single functioning kidney or significant bilateral disease [84, 85]. Nonoliguric renal failure has also been documented in children [86].

2. The renal systemic renin index has also been used to delineate patients with functional disease [46, 87]. It is calculated by subtracting the systemic PRA from the renal vein renin and dividing by the systemic PRA. A value greater than 0.48 documents a hemodynamically significant lesion, reflecting diminished renal blood flow.

3. A third ratio that can be checked is the contralateral renin suppression ratio. It is calculated by dividing the contralateral renal venous renin by the peripheral PRA. This ratio should be 1.3 or less.

TABLE 4.8
Formulae for Calculation of Renal Venous Renin Ratios

Formula	"Curability" Value
1. Lateralization $$\frac{\text{Ipsilateral renin}^a}{\text{Contralateral renin}^b}$$	≥1.5
2. Renal systemic renin index (Ipsilateral decreased renal plasma flow) $$\frac{\text{Ipsilateral renal vein renin} - \text{systemic PRA}}{\text{Systemic PRA}}$$	>0.48
3. Contralateral renal venous suppression $$\frac{\text{Contralateral renal venous renin}}{\text{Peripheral PRA}}$$	≤1.3

[a]Ipsilateral refers to the stenotic side.
[b]Contralateral refers to the nonstenotic side.

Thind [88] recommends the use of all three renal venous ratios described above for the most reliable prediction of renal ischemia (Table 4.8). He also recommends the use of a stimulated study, particularly in patients with bilateral stenosis, where the result can aid in the decision of which artery should be repaired first. It should be pointed out that despite all of the pitfalls inherent in renal vein renin determinations, they have a diagnostic accuracy of greater than 90% in children [35, 36, 89].

Arteriography can, however, be complicated by any of the following: (1) contrast-induced allergic reaction, (2) renal infarction (partial or complete) from the use of too large a catheter, (3) hematoma, (4) delayed hemorrhage, (5) thrombosis of the femoral artery used for access, and (5) minor emboli to the foot.

Doppler Ultrasound.   The Doppler ultrasound is a newer technique being evaluated for use as a potential screening tool for renovascular hypertension [90]. It has been suggested as a useful technique when linked to real-time ultrasound. The Doppler ultrasound occasionally fails to demonstrate a patent vessel lumen or Doppler blood flow [91, 92], but the latter does not necessarily give reliable evidence of arterial occlusion. However, the procedure is very time-consuming and is almost impossible to perform adequately in small children. This modality will require extensive evaluation in control trials with adults and children to determine its usefulness in assessing renovascular hypertension. Currently, it is still considered an experimental modality.

Renal Parenchymal Hypertension

Renal parenchymal diseases account for the majority of pediatric secondary hypertension cases. The most common etiology in this subgroup is interstitial nephritis or reflux nephropathy [93–95]. In adolescence, children affected with reflux nephropathy can have severe hypertension and encephalopathy without any perceived warning symptoms or elevations of BUN or creatinine. This disorder is usually associated with vesicoureteral reflux, though many children may have no history of documented recurrent urinary tract infection. This problem is most often bilateral with asymmetric disease. The more affected kidney is often smaller, and renal functional impairment varies from minimal to complete.

In the past, evaluation for possible chronic pyelonephritis has relied on the excretory urogram to demonstrate renal scarring. The scarring is demonstrated on intravenous pyelogram as focal parenchymal loss opposite a deformed calyx, giving the renal contour a lobulated irregular appearance. The images are essentially the same as those of the Ask-Upmark kidney [96], which was once thought to be a congenital segmental renal hypoplasia. Now it is actually thought to be a form of focal atrophic pyelonephritis [97, 98]. However, excretory urography does have some specific shortcomings. First, since adequate bowel preparation in children prior to study is often difficult, renal detail may be obscured by overlying bowel gas. Second, bony structures (ribs, spine in scoliosis) may obscure the renal image. In addition, an issue of particular concern is radiation dose to the gonads. Renal scintigraphy with either ^{99m}Tc-glucoheptonate or ^{99m}Tc-DMSA is very sensitive for detecting cortical scarring [99–101] and in many centers has replaced the excretory urogram. In fact, a large study in pediatric patients showed ^{99m}Tc-DMSA scanning to be significantly more sensitive, detecting several cases of pyelonephritic scarring before they were demonstrable by excretory urography [101]. The theoretical explanation put forth is that the functional abnormality, detected by scintigraphy, would occur immediately postinjury, but the anatomic abnormality (calyceal deformity and thinning parenchyma), detectable by excretory urogram, would take several months to develop. Additional advantages of this imaging technique include the fact that bowel gas or overlying bony structures do not affect the image, and radiation doses to the gonads are significantly less than those of excretory urography (because of radioisotope binding to renal tubular cells). Ultrasonography can assess renal size and contour, but there is debate about whether or not the level of sensitivity for detection of scars is actually better than that of excretory urography [102]. Despite this, renal ultrasound is often the first screening radiographic image, since no radiation is involved and differences in renal size can be accurately measured. The latter cannot be measured with scintigraphy, in which only relative differences can be noted. The other imaging study required in patients suspected of having chronic

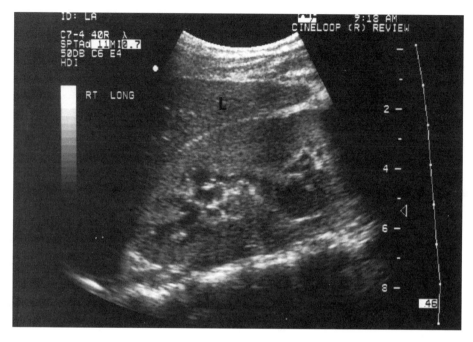

FIGURE 4.9. Increased echogenicity or "medical renal disease" is shown. The echogenicity of the kidney is similar to the liver (L). (Courtesy of Department of Radiology, Children's Hospital of Buffalo.)

pyelonephritis or pyelonephritic scarring is a voiding cystourethrogram, which is necessary because of the high association of chronic pyelonephritis with reflux nephropathy.

Chronic glomerulonephritis may also be associated with hypertension [95] (see Chapter 3). Both kidneys are always involved. Excretory urography or renal ultrasound demonstrate small kidneys. Renal ultrasound may show increased echogenicity (Figure 4.9) and occasionally calcifications. These etiologies are often associated with hematuria, proteinuria, and an abnormal urinary sediment (erythrocytes, leukocytes, or casts). In addition, an elevated BUN and creatinine, with other evidence of chronic renal insufficiency, may be present. However, definitive diagnosis usually requires a renal biopsy.

Papillary necrosis, from a variety of disease processes and toxic insults, can also be associated with hypertension. The common denominator is medullary ischemia resulting in elevated PRA. With papillary necrosis, excretory urography is the imaging study of choice. Excretory urography demonstrates central papillary cavitation with contrast extending into the medulla. Calcifications may also be noted. If the patient reaches end-stage disease, global atrophy, which is detectable by ultrasound, may result.

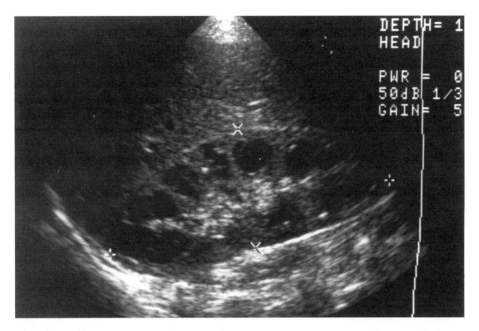

FIGURE 4.10. The renal sonogram shows markedly enlarged, echogenic kidneys with macrocystic changes sometimes observed in older children with autosomal recessive polycystic kidney disease. (Courtesy of Department of Radiology, Children's Hospital of Buffalo.)

The hypertension associated with autosomal recessive or autosomal dominant polycystic kidney disease (ARPKD or ADPKD) occurs at different points in the clinical course of the disease. The recessive form is most likely to come to attention because of palpable flank masses, with hypertension being a later finding. Hypertension may, however, be the sole presenting sign in the dominant form. Proteinuria, hematuria, and signs and symptoms of renal infection and lithiasis may occur concurrently in ADPKD. Family history is particularly important, especially for children in whom ADPKD may not be fully developed. Differentiation between ARPKD and ADPKD may be difficult initially in cases where there is no definitive family history. Ultrasonography is very important for initial screening [103–105]. In this screening, the recessive form demonstrates markedly enlarged, echogenic kidneys with macrocystic changes sometimes observed in older children (Figure 4.10). The dominant form shows large kidneys with multiple cysts of variable size in the cortex and medulla (Figure 4.11). One limitation of ultrasound in early ADPKD is its inability to detect cysts smaller than 1 cm in diameter. A computed tomographic (CT) scan has been used successfully for the diagnosis of both types of polycystic kidney disease [106–108] and is the preferred test for the defini-

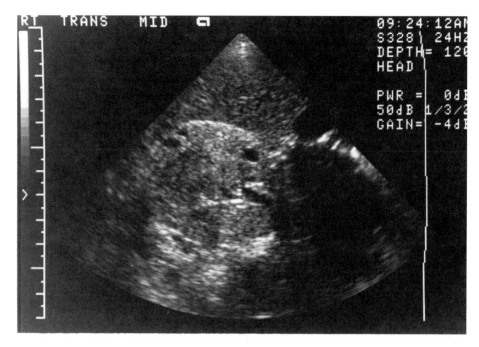

FIGURE 4.11. Autosomal dominant form of polycystic kidney disease shows large kidneys with multiple cysts of variable size in the cortex and medulla. (Courtesy of Department of Radiology, Children's Hospital of Buffalo.)

tive diagnosis of ADPKD [108]. An important advantage of this study over ultrasonography is its ability to reveal cysts smaller than 1 cm in diameter. In young children in whom the distinction between ARPKD and ADPKD is still not clear, liver and biliary tract ultrasonography may be helpful. These two methods can reveal either dilated ducts in ARPKD [109] or a cystic liver in ADPKD. However, in these uncertain cases, a liver and a renal biopsy are essential for definitive diagnosis of ARPKD [110]. The liver specimen in ARPKD reveals hepatic fibrosis and biliary dysgenesis.

Hydronephrosis with various etiologies may result in moderate to severe hypertension. Among these etiologies are ureteropelvic junction obstruction, ureterovesical obstruction, posterior urethral valves, ectopic ureterocele, and neurogenic bladder [111–115]. The diagnosis of hydronephrosis is made most easily by ultrasound. Bladder wall thickness can also be assessed using ultrasound. A voiding cystourethrogram should also be performed to determine whether the hydronephrosis is secondary to obstructive or nonobstructive dilatation. Renal function should be evaluated by renal scintigraphy (^{99m}Tc-DTPA). Renal scintigraphy can also differentiate functional from mechanical obstruction by using the furosemide washout technique [116] (Figure 4.12).

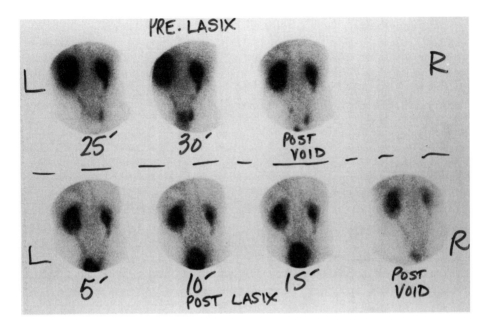

FIGURE 4.12. The upper panel shows limited excretion of the isotope. After the administration of furosemide (lower panel), there is increased excretion of the isotope. (Courtesy of Department of Radiology, Children's Hospital of Buffalo.)

Some renal and perirenal neoplasms are associated with hypertension, the most common of which is Wilms' tumor [117–119]. Despite this association, Wilms' tumor is unlikely to be detected solely because of hypertension. Evaluation is facilitated by a good physical examination, which reveals an abdominal mass. Both excretory urography and ultrasonography can demonstrate Wilms' tumor, but CT is needed for staging before definitive therapy. With a CT examination, one would see a well-defined, intrarenal soft-tissue mass distorting the collecting system. Calcifications may also be seen. The plasma renin activity can be elevated due to renal ischemia from renal artery compression or arteriovenous shunting within the tumor, or due to direct production of renin by the tumor [118–119].

Neuroblastoma may also result in hypertension, usually due to catecholamine hypersecretion. Increased renin may come into play if there is compression of the kidney or renal artery.

The Page kidney [120]—renal ischemia due to parenchymal compression by a perirenal hematoma—is a cause of hypertension that is best demonstrated by CT scan. There is enlargement of the affected kidney with a perirenal mass of fluid or soft tissue density.

Hemangiopericytoma is the final form of renal hypertension to be discussed. It is a very rare tumor that arises from juxtaglomerular cells, resulting in high-renin hypertension. It is usually detected by angiography in a patient being evaluated for renovascular hypertension [121]. If lateralization of renal venous renin ratios is detected but no lesion is noted on arteriogram, CT may demonstrate a small tumor.

Pheochromocytoma

Pheochromocytomas are rare, hormonally active tumors that produce hypertension by secreting norepinephrine and epinephrine. The patient's medical history is particularly helpful in these instances, with presenting complaints including headache, dizziness, weight loss, or increased appetite but failure to gain weight. There is also often a history of flushing, circumoral pallor, paroxysmal sweating, unexplained fevers, and palpitations. Occasionally, an asymptomatic patient may have a mass. On physical examination, hypertension and tachycardia, as well as postural hypotension, will be noted. These tumors may arise anywhere in the body where chromaffin tissue has occurred during development, but the most common site is in or near the adrenal glands. The diagnosis of pheochromocytoma should be particularly suspect in a perimenarchal girl with the above mentioned signs and symptoms.

The diagnosis of pheochromocytoma is usually confirmed by measurement of either increased catecholamines, their metabolites, or both in 24-hour urine and plasma renin activity (increased in about 70–80% of patients). The catecholamines and their metabolites include norepinephrine, epinephrine, dopamine, combined metanephrines, and vanillylmandelic acid (VMA). Normal urinary catecholamine catabolite values and factors that interfere with the urine measurements are given in Tables 4.9 and 4.10. If these values are normal but the diagnosis is still thought to be highly likely, the plasma norepinephrine and epinephrine levels should be checked. One large study showed the plasma catecholamines to be the single most reliable assay for determining the presence of pheochromocytoma [122]. If the plasma catecholamines are elevated but the clinical picture is questionable, an oral clonidine suppression test has proved to be useful in adults [123]. One 300-μg dose of oral clonidine causes a significant decrease in plasma norepinephrine levels three hours after ingestion in patients without pheochromocytoma. The plasma norepinephrine level is not suppressed if the patient has a secreting tumor. Currently, the dosage of clonidine to use for testing in children is not clear. If the urine or plasma catecholamine levels are found to be elevated, an abdominal CT scan should be obtained [124]. Contrast administration should only be done after alpha-blockade, because contrast may induce catecholamine release [125]. Because some pheochromocytoma tumors may be intrathoracic, CT examination of the chest should be performed if the abdominal study is

TABLE 4.9
Urinary Excretion of Vanillylmandelic Acid, Homovanillic Acid, and Total
Metanephrines in Children*

| Age (yrs) | Vanillylmandelic Acid | | Homovanillic Acid | | Total Metanephrines | |
	Mean	SD	Mean	SD	Mean	SD
<1	6.9	3.2	12.9	9.6	1.6	1.3
1–2	4.6	2.2	12.6	6.3	1.7	1.1
2–5	3.9	1.7	7.6	3.6	1.2	0.8
5–10	3.3	1.4	4.7	2.7	1.1	0.8
10–15	1.9	0.8	2.5	2.4	0.6	0.5
15–18	1.3	0.6	1.0	0.6	0.2	0.2

*All values are given as milligrams per milligram of creatinine.
Source: Reproduced with permission from SE Gitlow, M Mendlowitz, EK Wilk, et al. Excretion of catecholamine catabolites by normal children. J Lab Clin Med 1968;72:612.

negative. If the CT examination of the chest is also negative, scanning with ^{131}I-MIBG (metaiodobenzylguanidine), an analogue of norepinephrine which is selectively taken up by adrenergic tissue and concentrated in pheochromocytomas, should be used for diagnosis [126]. This has been shown to have the same sensitivity as CT scanning but has better specificity and allows the entire body to be imaged for primary or metastatic lesions [127]. This technique has not had an adequate trial in pediatric patients to advocate its use as a primary imaging mode [128]. If no tumor is located by MIBG scanning, the examiner should consider evaluation of the posterior cranial fossa, because some children can have astrocytoma, hypertension, and catecholamine excess [129]. In the past, angiography and vena caval sampling for catecholamines were used to localize pheochromocytoma. This practice is no longer necessary because newer diagnostic techniques are available. However, there are still times when angiography may be necessary, such as when encasement of major vessels is suspected.

Hyperaldosteronism

Primary hyperaldosteronism is rare in pediatrics, with adrenal hyperplasia occurring more frequently than adenoma. The former appears more frequently in boys and the latter is more common in girls. This disorder should be suspected in patients with a history of periodic muscular weakness and in whom preliminary laboratory evaluation reveals hypokalemic alkalosis and decreased PRA. These findings should prompt a check for elevated plasma aldosterone levels (Table 4.11). The hypokalemia is not always present, however, with up to 38% of adults with documented disease reported to have normal serum potassium levels [130]. It is important

TABLE 4.10
Factors That Interfere with Urine Tests for Catecholamines and Metabolites

Assay	Interfering Factors	
	Increase	*Decrease*
Catecholamines	**Pharmacologic**	**Pharmacologic**
	Exogenous catecholamines	Sympathetic nervous
	L-dopa, methyldopa	inhibitors (e.g., clonidine)
	Theophylline	Fenfluramine
	Analytic	Mendelamine (destroys
	Tetracycline, erythromycin	catecholamines in bladder
	Quinine, quinidine	urine)
	Chloral hydrate	
	Chlorpromazine	
	Labetalol	
Metanephrines	**Pharmacologic**	**Analytic**
	Exogenous catecholamines	Methylglucamine (radio-
	MAO inhibitors	graphic contrast)
	Rapid withdrawal of	Propranolol
	sympathetic inhibitors	
	Analytic	
	Acetaminophen	
	Benzodiazepines	
	Triamterene	
	Labetalol	
	Sotalol	
VMA	**Pharmacologic**	**Pharmacologic**
	Exogenous catecholamines	MAOIs
	L-dopa	Methyldopa
	Analytic	Ethanol
	Nalidixic acid	**Analytic**
	Anileridine	Clofibrate
	Disulfiram	Disulfiram
	Dietary phenolic acids (e.g.,	
	vanilla, bananas, coffee)	

MAOIs = monoamine oxidase inhibitors.
Source: Reproduced with permission from NM Kaplan. Pheochromocytoma. In NM Kaplan (ed), Clinical Hypertension. Baltimore: Williams & Wilkins, 1994;378.

to distinguish adenoma from hyperplasia because adenomas are amenable to surgical cure. Proposed laboratory tests to differentiate one from the other include measurement of overnight, recumbent 18-hydroxycorticosterone concentration and urinary 18-hydroxycortisol levels [131–133]. The diagnostic imaging study of choice is a CT scan, revealing bilateral adrenal

TABLE 4.11
Normal Values for Pediatric Plasma Aldosterone Levels

Age	Median in ng/dl (range)
1 wk–3 mos	62 (30–201)
3–12 mos	18 (7–39)
1–4 yrs	15 (3–77)
4–8 yrs	11 (5–20)
8–13 yrs	8 (4–17)

Source: Modified from TJW Fiselier, P Lijnen, L Monnens, et al. Levels of renin, angiotensin I and II, angiotensin-converting enzyme, and aldosterone in infancy and childhood. Eur J Pediatr 1983;141:3.

enlargement in the case of hyperplasia and a unilateral, well-defined, homogeneous mass in the case of adenoma. Ultrasonography has the disadvantage of being unable to detect smaller lesions. An investigational radiopharmaceutical, ^{131}I iodonorcholesterol, requires an extensive examination time (4–15 days) and dexamethasone suppression and requires a high radiation dose [65].

Glucocorticoid-remediable aldosteronism (GRA) is an autosomal dominant disorder that can result in childhood hypertension [134]. The family history is particularly important in these cases, as one usually finds a history of early-onset hypertension in many relatives. In these cases, the usually low PRA increases in response to dexamethasone. This fact can be used in the diagnostic work-up. There is a direct genetic blood test for detecting GRA. Information about the genetic blood tests for detecting GRA is available from the International Registry for Glucocorticoid-Remediable Aldosteronism [800-GRA-2262 (Robert Dluhy, Brigham and Women's Hospital, Boston; Richard Lifton, Yale University, New Haven)].

Cushing's Disease

Cushing's disease, which is due to endogenous cortisol production, is a very rare cause of childhood hypertension. Hypertension secondary to administration of exogenous corticosteroids commonly occurs. The history and physical examination of children with Cushing's disease are usually very striking—weight gain, easy bruising, truncal obesity, moon facies, striae, hirsutism, and a buffalo hump. Preliminary laboratory evaluation will reveal glucosuria and hyperglycemia. Specific laboratory tests used to diagnose Cushing's disease include a search for increased plasma cortisol and increased urinary excretion of 17-hydroxycorticoids. The classic test used to make this diagnosis has been the dexamethasone suppression test. This relies on the fact that 1 mg of exogenous dexamethasone given at 11 P.M. should inhibit the normal early morning (2 A.M.)

outflow of adrenocorticotropic hormone (ACTH) from the pituitary gland, thus preventing the normal rise of plasma cortisol levels to their maximum at 6 A.M. In the case of Cushing's disease, the cortisol levels are not suppressed after the dose of dexamethasone, because the elevated levels in these instances are independent of ACTH secretion.

Children with Severe Hypertension

The most important fact to keep in mind about children with severe hypertension is that treatment takes precedence over evaluation. A thorough evaluation can be undertaken after the BP is safely out of critical range. The majority of these children have renal or endocrinologic causes for their hypertension, though some will be diagnosed as essential hypertensives. As indicated in the previous section, the work-up in these children should initially proceed as dictated by the history, physical examination, and preliminary laboratory data. In general, these children require an extensive search for a hypertensive etiology, before they are labeled as essential hypertensives.

Children with Chronic Hypertension

Unless serial BPs are available over an extended period of time, the chronicity of hypertension in the pediatric age group cannot be established. In many cases, the major indicator of chronicity is the presence of end- or target-organ damage. The presence, or absence, of target-organ damage is also often used to determine whether to initiate pharmacologic treatment in children with mild to moderate BP elevations. The three organs to which the term target-organ applies are the eye, heart, and kidney.

Examination by an ophthalmologist is absolutely indicated in patients with known chronic hypertension, or those in whom the duration of hypertension is uncertain. The ophthalmologist will be able to detect mild funduscopic changes that may be missed by the nonophthalmologist. The classic findings of hemorrhages and exudates described in adults are rare in the pediatric age group. Often the only findings, if any, are arteriolar narrowing and arteriovenous thickening. These changes are not reversible, but their progression may be slowed or prevented by early intervention and control of BP.

Abnormal values of BUN, creatinine, or uric acid may provide evidence of renal damage. These values should be obtained in the initial screening laboratory test of a hypertensive child. An elevated BUN and creatinine may be indicative of either renal damage secondary to longstanding hypertension or a renal etiology for the hypertension. A uric acid measurement may be helpful, because it may be elevated in chronic hypertension before more overt evidence of renal functional impairment (such as elevated BUN or creatinine) is present [27, 28].

Concentric hypertrophy of the left ventricular muscle is thought to be the response of the heart to the increased pressure load produced by hypertension [135]. As with hypertensive adults, hypertensive pediatric patients are prone to develop left ventricular hypertrophy (LVH) [136, 137]. The prevalence of LVH in pediatric hypertensive patients has been reported at 11.0–38.5%, depending on the population studied and method used to assess cardiac enlargement [138–140]. Of importance, however, is the fact that the level and duration of elevated BP are not the only precipitating factors [141]. In addition to average systolic BP, other variables that seem to indicate a predisposition to develop LVH include male sex [140, 142, 143], body mass index [140, 144, 145], and sodium intake [140, 146–148]. The detection of LVH is particularly important because of the associated morbidity and mortality. The Framingham study showed that hypertensive adults with LVH had a 10-fold greater risk of developing congestive heart failure when compared to those without LVH [149]. Another study showed LVH, in and of itself, to be a risk factor for cardiovascular morbidity and mortality [150]. Early intervention to control hypertension may result in reversal of the hypertrophy, which in turn would decrease the associated morbidity.

The chest x-ray has not been shown to be a sensitive method for detection of LVH, and the electrocardiogram has a tendency to give false-positive results in children [151]. Echocardiography has the advantage of being a noninvasive method that allows the direct measurement of cardiac dimensions and wall thickness [152]. From these values, left ventricular mass can be calculated. One important study showed that echocardiography is the most sensitive method for detecting myocardial hypertrophy [138]. It is significant that LVH may be present in adolescents with only mild, persistent hypertension [138], and even those with only borderline hypertension [139]. This clearly indicates that one should not rely on the level of hypertension to determine when to check for target-organ damage.

Summary

Evaluation of pediatric hypertension can be an extremely prolonged and expensive venture, if the program is not tailored to the individual child (Figure 4.13). The importance of a thorough history and physical examination cannot be overstated. These in combination with some basic laboratory studies should give some insight into possible etiologies. The rare endocrinologic causes of hypertension in children will generally have very specific findings, and it is therefore not necessary to evaluate every hypertensive child for endocrinologic abnormalities. The lack of specific indicators from the preliminary work-up, especially in a very young child or one

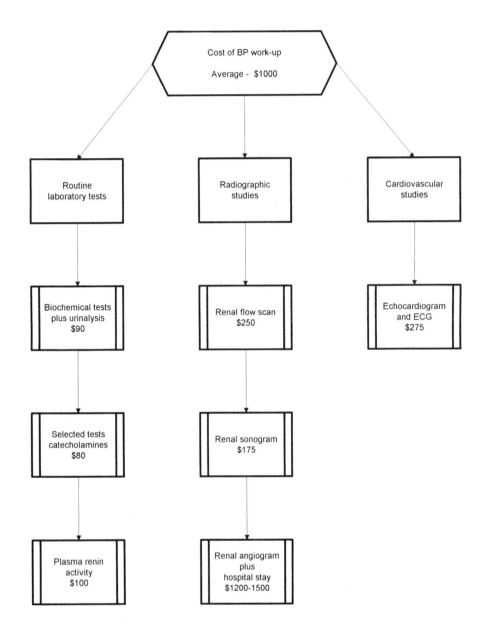

FIGURE 4.13. Average costs of a limited hypertensive work-up.

with severe hypertension, should not preclude a search for a renal etiology, since this will be the most frequent finding after essential hypertension. Essential hypertension, though the most common diagnosis, should remain a diagnosis of exclusion.

References

1. Dillon MJ. Investigation and management of hypertension in children. A personal perspective. Pediatr Nephrol 1987;1:59.
2. Loggie JMH. Evaluation and management of childhood hypertension. Surg Clin North Am 1985;65:1623.
3. Ogborn MR, Crocker JFS. Investigation of pediatric hypertension. Use of a tailored protocol. Am J Dis Child 1987;141:1205.
4. Loggie JMH. Hypertension in children and adolescents. Hosp Pract (Off Ed) 1975;10:81.
5. Task Force on Blood Pressure Control in Children. Report of the Second Task Force on Blood Pressure Control in Children—1987. Pediatrics 1987;79:1.
6. Gillum RF, Prineas RJ, Horibe H. Maturation vs age: assessing blood pressure by height. J Natl Med Assoc 1982;74:43.
7. Portman RJ, Lugo-Miro VI, Ikle D, et al. Diagnosis of adolescent hypertension on initial screening by the use of height age. J Adol Health Care 1990;11:215.
8. Prineas RJ, Gillum RF, Horibe H. The Minneapolis Children's Blood Pressure Study. Part 2: Multiple determinants of children's blood pressure. Hypertension 1980;2:I25.
9. Harlan WR, Corroni-Huntley J, Leaverton PE. Blood pressure in childhood: The National Health Examination Survey. Hypertension 1979;1:559.
10. Voors AW, Webber LS, Frerichs RR, et al. Body height and body mass as determinants of basal blood pressure in children—the Bogalusa Heart Study. Am J Epidemiol 1977;106:101.
11. Lauer RM, Clarke WR, Beaglehole R. Level, trend and variability of blood pressure during childhood: The Muscatine Study. Circulation 1984;69:242.
12. Voors AW, Webber LS, Berenson GS. A consideration of essential hypertension in children. Pract Cardiol 1977;3:29.
13. Katz SH, Hediger ML, Schall JI, et al. Blood pressure, growth and maturation from childhood through adolescence. Mixed longitudinal analyses of the Philadelphia Blood Pressure Project. Hypertension 1980;2:155.
14. Pickering TG, Harshfield GA, Kleinert HD, et al. BP during normal daily activities, sleep and exercise—comparison of values in normal and hypertensive subjects. JAMA 1982;247:992.
15. Mancia G, Bertinieri G, Grassi G, et al. Effects of blood pressure measurement by the doctor on patient's blood pressure and heart rate. Lancet 1983;2:695.
16. Perloff D, Sokolow M, Cowan R. The prognostic value of ambulatory blood pressures. JAMA 1983;249:2792.
17. Di Renzo M, Grassi G, Pedotti A, et al. Continuous versus intermittent blood pressure measurement in estimating 24-hour average blood pressure. Hypertension 1983;5:264.
18. Brunner HR, Coombs BJ, Waeber B, et al. Accuracy and reproducibility of ambulatory blood pressure recordings obtained with the Remler system. J Hypertens 1983;1:291.

19. Pickering TG, Harshfield GA, Devereux L, et al. What is the role of ambulatory blood pressure monitoring in the management of hypertensive patients? Hypertension 1985;7:171.

20. Conway J, Johnston J, Coates A, et al. The use of ambulatory blood pressure monitoring to improve the accuracy and reduce the number of subjects in clinical trials of antihypertensive agents. J Hypertens 1988;6:111.

21. Parati G, Pomidossi G, Albini F, et al. Relationship of 24-hour blood pressure mean and variability to severity of target organ damage in hypertension. J Hypertens 1987;5:93.

22. Sokolow M, Werdegar D, Kain H, et al. Relationship between level of blood pressure measured casually and by portable recorders and severity of complications in essential hypertension. Circulation 1966;34:279.

23. Rowlands DB, Ireland MA, Glover DR, et al. The relationship between ambulatory blood pressure and electrocardiographically assessed left ventricular hypertrophy. Clin Sci 1981;61(Suppl 7):101.

24. Lloyd AVC, Jewitt DE, Still JDL. Facial paralysis in children with hypertension. Arch Dis Child 1966;41:292.

25. Siegler RL, Brewer ED, Corneli HM. Hypertension first seen as facial paralysis: case reports and review of the literature. Pediatrics 1991;87:387.

26. Prebis JW, Gruskin AB, Polinsky MS. Uric acid in childhood essential hypertension. J Pediatr 1981;98:702.

27. Messerli FH, Frohlich ED, Dreslinski GR et al. Serum uric acid in essential hypertension: an indicator of renal vascular involvement. Ann Intern Med 1980;93:817.

28. Hiner LB, Gruskin AB, Baluarte HJ, et al. Plasma renin activity in normal children. J Pediatr 1976;89:258.

29. Sassard J, Sann L, Vincent M, et al. Plasma renin activity in normal subjects from infancy to puberty. J Clin Endocrinol Metab 1975;40:524.

30. Stalker HP, Holland NH, Kotchen JM, et al. Plasma renin activity in healthy children. J Pediatr 1976;89:256.

31. Fiselier TJW, Lijnen P, Monnens L, et al. Levels of renin, angiotensin I and II, angiotensin-converting enzyme and aldosterone in infancy and childhood. Eur J Pediatr 1983;141:3.

32. Goldberg S, Krishan I, Hames CB, et al. Elevated renin levels in normotensive adolescents. Pediatrics 1974;54:596.

33. Bauer JH, Sunderrajan S, Reams G. Effects of calcium entry blockers on renin-angiotensin–aldosterone system, renal function and hemodynamics, salt and water excretion and body fluid composition. Am J Cardiol 1985;56:62.

34. Fry WJ, Ernst CB, Stanley JC, et al. Renovascular hypertension in the pediatric patient. Arch Surg 1973;107:692.

35. Lawson JD, Boerth R, Foster JH, et al. Diagnosis and management of renovascular hypertension in children. Arch Surg 1977;112:1307.

36. Stanley P, Gyepes MT, Olson DL, et al. Renovascular hypertension in children and adolescents. Radiology 1978;129:123.

37. Krorbkin M, Perloff DL, Palubinskas AJ. Renal arteriography in the evaluation of unexplained hypertension in children and adolescents. J Pediatr 1976;88:388.
38. Ernst CB. Childhood Renovascular Hypertension. In TA Kotchen, JM Kotchen (eds), High Blood Pressure in the Young. Littleton, MA: John Wright-PSG, 1983;151.
39. Adelman RD. Neonatal hypertension. Pediatr Clin North Am 1978;25:99.
40. Muller FB, Sealey JE, Case DB, et al. The captopril test for identifying renovascular disease in hypertensive patients. Am J Med 1986;80:633.
41. Gaul MK, Linn WD, Mulrow CD. Captopril stimulated renin secretion in the diagnosis of renovascular hypertension. Am J Hypertens 1989;2:335.
42. Gosse P, Dupas JY, Reynaud P, et al. The captopril test in the detection of renovascular hypertension in a population with low prevalence of the disease. A prospective study. Am J Hypertens 1989;2:191.
43. Willems CED, Shah V, Uchiyama M, et al. The captopril test: an aid to investigation of hypertension. Arch Dis Child 1989;64:229.
44. Gauthier B, Trachtman H, Frank R, et al. Inadequacy of captopril challenge test for diagnosing renovascular hypertension in children and adolescents. Pediatr Nephrol 1991;5:42.
45. Bookstein JJ, Abrams HL, Buenger RE, et al. Cooperative study of renovascular hypertension. Radiologic aspects of renovascular hypertension. Part 2. The role of urography in unilateral renovascular disease. JAMA 1972;220:1225.
46. Stanley JC, Fry WJ. Pediatric renal artery occlusive disease and renovascular hypertension. Arch Surg 1981;116:669.
47. Bookstein JJ, Maxwell MH, Abrams HL, et al. Cooperative study of radiologic aspects of renovascular hypertension. JAMA 1977;237:1706.
48. Arlat I, Rosenthal J, Adam WE, et al. Predictive value of radionuclide methods in the diagnosis of unilateral renovascular hypertension. Cardiovasc Radiol 1979;2:115.
49. Chiarini C, Esposti ED, Losinno F, et al. Renal scintigraphy versus renal vein renin for identifying and treating renovascular hypertension. Nephron 1982;32:8.
50. Rosen PR, Treves S, Ingelfinger J. Hypertension in children. Increased efficacy of technetium Tc 99m succimer in screening for renal disease. Am J Dis Child 1985;139:173.
51. Geyskes GG, Oei HY, Puylaert AJ. Renography with captopril: changes in a patient with hypertension and unilateral renal artery stenosis. Arch Intern Med 1986;146:1705.
52. Fommei E, Ghione S, Palla L, et al. Renal scintigraphic captopril test in the diagnosis of renovascular hypertension. Hypertension 1987;10:212.
53. Sfakianakis GN, Bourgoignie JJ, Jaffe D, et al. Single-dose captopril scintigraphy in the diagnosis of renovascular hypertension. J Nucl Med 1987;28:1383.
54. Meier GH, Sumpio B, Black HR, et al. Captopril renal scintigraphy—an advance in the detection and treatment of renovascular hypertension. J Vasc Surg 1990;11:770.

55. Majd M, Potter BM, Guzzetta PC, et al. Captopril enhanced renal scintigraphy for detection of renal artery stenosis—an update [abstract]. J Nucl Med 1986;27:962.

56. Daly MJ, Henry RE. Defining renal anatomy and function with Tc-99m DMSA: clinical and renographic correlation. J Urol 1981;126:5.

57. Vivian G, Stringer D, de Bruyn R, et al. Tc-99m DMSA in Renovascular Hypertension in Children. In C Raynaud (ed), Proceedings of the Third World Congress of Nuclear Medicine and Biology, Vol 4. Paris: Pergamon Press, 1982;2663.

58. Oppenheimer DA, Carroll BA, Garth KE. Ultrasonic detection of complications following umbilical arterial catheterization in the neonate. Radiology 1982;145:667.

59. Rosenfeild AT, Zeman RK, Cronan JJ, et al. Ultrasound in experimental and clinical renal vein thrombosis. Radiology 1980;137:735.

60. Hillman BJ. Digital radiology of the kidney. Radiol Clin North Am 1985;23:211.

61. Zabbo A, Novick AC. Digital subtraction angiography for noninvasive imaging of the renal artery. Urol Clin North Am 1984;11:409.

62. Havey RJ, Krumlovsky F, delGreco F, et al. Screening for renovascular hypertension. Is renal digital subtraction angiography the preferred noninvasive test? JAMA 1985;254:388.

63. Amundson GM, Wesenberg RL, Mueller DL, et al. Pediatric digital subtraction angiography. Radiology 1984;153:649.

64. Buonocore E, Meaney TF, Borkowski GP, et al. Digital subtraction angiography in the abdominal aorta and renal arteries. Comparison with conventional angiography. Radiology 1981;139:281.

65. Siegel MJ, St Amour TE, Siegel BA. Imaging techniques in the evaluation of pediatric hypertension. Pediatr Nephrol 1987;1:76.

66. Foley WD, Milde MW. Intra-arterial digital subtraction angiography. Radiol Clin North Am 1985;23:293.

67. Stringer DA, de Bruyn R, Dillon MJ. Comparison of aortography, renal vein renin sampling, radionuclide scans, ultrasound and the IVU in the investigation of childhood renovascular hypertension. Br J Radiol 1984;57:111.

68. Mena E, Bookstein JJ, Holt JF, et al. Neurofibromatosis and renovascular hypertension in children. AJR Am J Roentgenol 1973;118:39.

69. Greene JF Jr, Fitzwater JE, Burgess J. Arterial lesions associated with neurofibromatosis. Am J Clin Pathol 1974;62:481.

70. Kirks DR, Fitz CR, Korobkin M. Intrarenal collateral circulation in the pediatric patient. Pediatr Radiol 1977;5:154.

71. Eyler WR, Clark MD, Garman JE, et al. Angiography of the renal areas including a comparative study of renal arterial stenoses in patients with and without hypertension. Radiology 1962;78:879.

72. Holley KE, Hunt JC, Brown AL, et al. Renal artery stenosis: a clinical-pathological study in normotensive patients. Am J Med 1964;37:14.

73. Marks LS, Maxwell MH, Renal vein renin value and limitation in the prediction of operative results. Urol Clin North Am 1975;2:311.

74. Korobkin M, Glickman MG, Schambelan M. Segmental renal vein sampling for renin. Radiology 1976;118:307.
75. Mannick JA, Huvos A, Hollander WE. Post-hydralazine renin release in the diagnosis of renovascular hypertension. Ann Surg 1969;170:409.
76. Gittes RF, McLaughlin AP III. Unilateral operation for bilateral renovascular disease. J Urol 1974;111:292.
77. Gomes AS, Sinaiko AR, Tobian L, et al. Hydralazine and the tourniquet test in renal vein renin sampling: a comparison. Radiology 1983;146:657.
78. Thind GS, Montojo PM, Johnson A, et al. Enhancement of renal venous renin ratios by intravenous hydralazine in renovascular hypertension. Am J Cardiol 1984;53:109.
79. Kaneko Y, Ikeda T, Takeda T, et al. Renin release during acute reduction of arterial pressure in normotensive subjects and patients with renovascular hypertension. J Clin Invest 1967;46:705.
80. Stokes GS, Weber MA, Gain M, et al. Diazoxide-induced renin release in diagnosis of remediable renovascular hypertension. Aust N Z J Med 1976;6:26.
81. Lyons DF, Streck WF, Kem DC, et al. Captopril stimulation of differential renins in renovascular hypertension. Hypertension 1983;5:615.
82. Thibonnier M, Joseph A, Sassano P, et al. Improved diagnosis of unilateral renal artery lesions after captopril administration. JAMA 1984;251:56.
83. Tomoda F, Takata M, Ohashi S, et al. Captopril-stimulated renal vein renin in hypertensive patients with or without renal artery stenosis. Am J Hypertens 1990;3:918.
84. Hricik DE, Browning PJ, Kopelman R, et al. Captopril-induced functional renal insufficiency in patients with bilateral renal artery stenosis or renal artery stenosis in a solitary kidney. N Engl J Med 1983;308:373.
85. Chrysant SG, Dunn M, Marples D, et al. Severe reversible azotemia from captopril therapy: report of three cases and review of the literature. Arch Intern Med 1983;143:437.
86. Colavita RD, Gaudio KM, Siegel NJ. Reversible reduction in renal function during treatment with captopril. Pediatrics 1983;71:839.
87. Sealey JE, Buhler FR, Laragh JH, et al. The physiology of renin secretion in essential hypertension: estimation of renin secretion rate and renal plasma flow from peripheral and renal vein renin levels. Am J Med 1973;55:391.
88. Thind GS. Role of renal venous renins in the diagnosis and management of renovascular hypertension. J Urol 1985;134:2.
89. Kaufman JJ, Goodwin WE, Waisman JJ, et al. Renovascular hypertension in children: report of seven cases treated surgically including two cases of renal autotransplantation. Am J Surg 1972;24:149.
90. Taylor DC, Kettler MD, Moneta GL, et al. Duplex ultrasound scanning in the diagnosis of renal artery stenosis: a prospective evaluation. J Vasc Surg 1988;7:363.
91. Greene ER, Venters MD, Avasthi PA. Non-invasive characterization of renal artery blood flow. Kidney Int 1981;20:523.

92. Dubbins PA. Renal artery stenosis: duplex Doppler evaluation. Br J Radiol 1986;59:225.
93. Rance CP, Arbus GS, Balfe JW, et al. Persistent systemic hypertension in infants and children. Pediatr Clin North Am 1974;21:801.
94. Holland NH, Kotchen T, Bhathena D. Hypertensive children with chronic pyelonephritis. Kidney Int 1975;8:243.
95. Gill DG, da Costa BM, Cameron JS, et al. Analysis of 100 children with severe and persistent hypertension. Arch Dis Child 1976;51:951.
96. Himmelfarb E, Rabinowitz JG, Parvey L, et al. The Ask-Upmark kidney: roentgenographic and pathological features. Am J Dis Child 1975;129:1440.
97. Arant BS Jr, Sotelo-Avita C, Berstein J. Segmental "hypoplasia" of the kidney (Ask-Upmark). J Pediatr 1979;95:931.
98. Shindo S, Berstein J, Arant BS Jr. Evolution of renal segmental atrophy (Ask-Upmark kidney) in children with vesicoureteric reflux: radiographic and morphologic studies. J Pediatr 1983;102:847.
99. McAfee JG. Radionuclide imaging in the assessment of primary chronic pyelonephritis. Radiology 1979;133:203.
100. Merrick MV, Uttley WS, Wild SR. The detection of pyelonephritic scarring in children by radioisotope scanning. Br J Radiol 1980;53:544.
101. Kogan BA, Kay R, Wasnick RJ. ^{99m}Tc-DMSA scanning to diagnose pyelonephritic scarring in children. Urology 1983;21:641.
102. Leonidas JC, McCauley RGK, Klauber GC, et al. Sonography as a substitute for excretory urography in children with urinary tract infection. AJR Am J Roentgenol 1985;144:815.
103. Boal DK, Teele RL. Sonography of infantile polycystic kidney disease. AJR Am J Roentgenol 1980;135:575.
104. Grossman H, Rosenberg ER, Bowie JD, et al. Sonographic diagnosis of renal cystic diseases. AJR Am J Roentgenol 1983;140:81.
105. Sedman A, Bell P, Manco-Johnson M, et al. Autosomal dominant polycystic kidney disease in childhood: a longitudinal study. Kidney Int 1987;31:1000.
106. Howie JL, Nicholson RL. CT evaluation of infantile polycystic disease. J Can Assoc Radiol 1980;31:202.
107. Berger PE, Munschauer RW, Kuhn JP. Computed tomography and ultrasound of renal and perirenal diseases in infants and children. Pediatr Radiol 1980;9:91.
108. Levine E, Grantham JJ. The role of computed tomography in the evaluation of adult polycystic kidney disease. Am J Kidney Dis 1981;1:99.
109. Marchal GJ, Desmet VJ, Proesmans WC, et al. Caroli disease: high frequency US and pathologic findings. Radiology 1986;158:507.
110. Cole BR, Conley SB, Stapleton FB. Polycystic kidney disease in the first year of life. J Pediatr 1987;111:693.
111. Nemoy NJ, Fichman MP, Sellers A. Unilateral ureteral obstruction. A cause of reversible high renin content hypertension. JAMA 1973;225:512.
112. Schiff M Jr, McGuire EJ, Baskin AM. Hypertension and unilateral hydronephrosis. Urology 1975;5:178.

113. Vaughan ED Jr, Buhler FR, Laragh JH, et al. Hypertension and unilateral parenchymal renal disease. JAMA 1975;233:1177.

114. Grossman IC, Cromie WJ, Wein AJ, et al. Renal hypertension secondary to ureteropelvic junction obstruction. Unusual presentation and new therapeutic modality. Urology 1981;17:69.

115. Riehle RA, Vaughan ED. Renin participation in hypertension associated with unilateral hydronephrosis. J Urol 1981;120:243.

116. Ash JM, Antico VF, Gilday DL, et al. Special considerations in the pediatric use of radionuclides in kidney studies. Semin Nucl Med 1982;12:345.

117. Hughes JH, Rosenblum H, Horn LG. Hypertension in embryoma (Wilm's tumor). Pediatrics 1949;3:201.

118. Ganguly A, Gribble J, Tune B. Renin-secreting Wilm's tumor with severe hypertension. Report of a case and brief review of renin secreting tumors. Ann Intern Med 1973;79:835.

119. Spahr J, Demers LMN, Shochat SJ. Renin producing Wilm's tumor. J Pediatr Surg 1981;16:32.

120. Page IH. The production of persistent arterial hypertension by cellophane perinephritis. JAMA 1939;113:2046.

121. Conn JM, Bookstein JJ, Cohen EL. Renin-secreting juxtaglomerular cell adenoma. Preoperative clinical and angiographic diagnosis. Radiology 1973;106:543.

122. Bravo EL, Tarazi RC, Gifford RW, et al. Circulating and urinary catecholamines in pheochromocytoma. Diagnostic and pathophysiologic implications. N Engl J Med 1979;301:682.

123. Bravo EL, Tarazi RC, Fouad FM, et al. Clonodine-suppression test. A useful aid in the diagnosis of pheochromocytoma. N Engl J Med 1981;305:623.

124. Stewart BH, Bravo EL, Haaga J, et al. Localization of pheochromocytoma by CT scan. N Engl J Med 1978;299:460.

125. Raisanen J, Shapiro B, Glazer GM, et al. Plasma catecholamines in pheochromocytoma. Effect of urographic contrast media. Am J Radiol 1984;143:43.

126. Sisson JC, Frager MS, Valk TW, et al. Scintigraphic location of pheochromocytoma. N Engl J Med 1981;305:12.

127. Francis IR, Glazer GM, Shapiro B, et al. Complementary roles of CT and ^{131}I-MIBG scintigraphy in diagnosing pheochromocytoma. AJR Am J Roentgenol 1983;141:719.

128. Quint LE, Glazer GM, Francis IR, et al. Pheochromocytoma and paraganglioma: comparison of MR imaging with CT and I-131 MIBG scintigraphy. Radiology 1987;165:89.

129. Evans CH, Westfall V, Atuk N. Astrocytoma mimicking the features of pheochromocytoma. N Engl J Med 1972;286:1397.

130. Ferris JB, Beevers DG, Brown J. Clinical, biochemical and pathological features of low-renin (primary) hyperaldosteronism. Am Heart J 1978;95:375.

131. Biglieri EG, Schambelan M. The significance of elevated levels of plasma 18-hydroxycorticosterone in patients with primary aldosteronism. J Clin Endocrinol Metab 1979;48:87.

132. Bravo EL, Tarazi RC, Dustan HP, et al. The changing clinical spectrum of primary aldosteronism. Am J Med 1983;74:641.

133. Ulick S, Chu MD. Hypersecretion of a new corticosteroid, 18-hydroxycortisol, in two types of adrenocortical hypertension. J Clin Exp Hypertens 1982; A4:1771.

134. New MI, Oberfield SE, Levine LS, et al. Demonstration of autosomal dominant transmission and absence of HLA linkage in dexamethasone suppressible hyperaldosteronism. Lancet 1980;1:550.

135. Grossman W, Jones D, McLaurin LP. Wall stress and patterns of hypertrophy in human left ventricle. J Clin Invest 1975;56:56.

136. Laird WP, Fixler DE. Hypertension in adolescents: an ultrasound study. Ultrasound Med Biol 1976;2:49.

137. Schieken RM, Clarke WR, Lauer RM. Left ventricular hypertrophy in children with blood pressures in the upper quintile of the distribution. The Muscatine study. Hypertension 1981;3:669.

138. Laird WP, Fixler DE. Left ventricular hypertrophy in adolescents with elevated blood pressure: assessment by chest roentgenography, electrocardiography and echocardiography. Pediatrics 1981;67:255.

139. Culpepper WS III, Sodt PG, Messerli FH, et al. Cardiac status in juvenile borderline hypertension. Ann Intern Med 1983;98:1.

140. Daniels SD, Meyer RA, Loggie JMH. Determinants of cardiac involvement in children and adolescents with essential hypertension. Circulation 1990;82:1243.

141. Drayer J, Gardin J, Brewer D, et al. Disparate relationships between blood pressure and left ventricular mass in patients with and without left ventricular hypertrophy. Hypertension 1987;9:161.

142. Daniels SR, Meyer RA, Liang YC, et al. Echocardiography determined left ventricular mass index in normal children, adolescents and young adults. J Am Coll Cardiol 1988;12:703.

143. Burke GL, Arcilla RA, Culpepper WS, et al. Blood pressure and echocardiographic measures in children: the Bogalusa Heart Study. Circulation 1987;5:106.

144. Hammond IW, Devereux RB, Alderman MH, et al. Relationship of blood pressure and body build to left ventricular mass in normotensive and hypertensive employed adults. J Am Coll Cardiol 1988;12:996.

145. MacMahon SW, Wilcken DEL, Macdonald GJ. The effect of weight reduction on left ventricular mass: a randomized control trial in young overweight hypertensive patients. N Engl J Med 1986;314:334.

146. Lindpainter K, Sen S. Role of sodium in hypertensive cardiac hypertrophy. Circ Res 1985;57:610.

147. Schmeider RE, Messerli FJ, Garavaglia GE, et al. Dietary salt intake: a determinant of cardiac involvement in essential hypertension. Circulation 1988;8:951.

148. Ferrara LA, DeSimone G, Pasanisi F, et al. Left ventricular mass reduction during salt depletion in arterial hypertension. Hypertension 1987;6:755.

149. Kannel WB, Castelli WP, McNamara PM, et al. Role of blood pressure in the development of congestive heart failure: the Framingham Study. N Engl J Med 1972;287:781.

150. Casale PN, Devereux RB, Milner M, et al. Value of echocardiographic measurement of left ventricular mass in predicting cardiovascular morbid events in hypertensive men. Ann Intern Med 1986;105:173.

151. Morganroth J, Maron BJ, Krovetz LJ, et al. Electrocardiographic evidence of left ventricular hypertrophy in otherwise normal children: classification by echocardiography. Am J Cardiol 1975;35:278.

152. Troy BL, Pombo J, Rackley CE. Measurement of left ventricular wall thickness and mass by echocardiography. Circulation 1972;45:602.

CHAPTER 5

Nonpharmacologic Therapy of Hypertension

Leonard G. Feld and Wayne R. Waz

The possibility of treating hypertension without medications is appealing. The prospect of a lifetime of daily medication can be discouraging, particularly for children and adolescents with hypertension. Although pharmacologic therapy has undergone remarkable advances in recent years, side effects, adverse reactions, and costs have not been eliminated. An important consideration in the use of any antihypertensive therapy (including nonpharmacologic measures) is whether the side effects are tolerable in light of the severity of the disease. Treatment of hypertension is often complicated by poor compliance: Many patients find it difficult to follow a regimen that seldom improves (and often diminishes) their quality of life over the short term. The lack of perceived gain that deters compliance is particularly worrisome (although not unique) in adolescents, who may find discussions of heart disease, stroke, and renal insufficiency to be abstract and irrelevant.

This chapter addresses nonpharmacologic interventions that may help to reduce blood pressure (BP). Many of the interventions involve lifestyle modifications that, like medications, alter a patient's daily routine. An important component in the initiation and subsequent success of any therapy—be it medication, sodium restriction, weight loss, or any of the other interventions discussed below—is an ongoing dialogue between the physician and the patient and/or parents. In cases warranting antihypertensive therapy, patients rarely feel ill, yet are asked to follow a daily regimen for an indefinite period of time. Families need to be aware of the rationale behind such antihypertensive therapy.

TABLE 5.1
Nonpharmacologic Therapy of Hypertension

Sodium restriction
Potassium, calcium, and magnesium supplements
Weight loss
Exercise
Lifestyle modification (i.e., alcohol, cigarettes, stress)

Table 5.1 lists several nonpharmacologic therapies that have been used in the treatment of hypertension. In this chapter, each of these areas is reviewed with recommendations regarding their use, both as primary therapies and as adjuncts to medications.

Salt Restriction

The relationship between salt intake (primarily sodium chloride) and BP has been studied extensively since the beginning of this century [1], yet no definitive mechanism for the hypertensive effect of a high-sodium diet has been elucidated. Because of the lack of a well-defined mechanism, sodium restriction remains controversial. However, in discussions of antihypertensive therapy most authors recommend some form of salt restriction [2–5]. This section reviews both human and animal studies of the relationship between salt and BP, with particular emphasis on studies involving children. We address two major areas: (1) identification of "salt-sensitive" individuals in whom sodium restriction may be particularly effective, and (2) recommendations on the use of salt restriction.

Studies in humans can be divided into 3 groups: (1) studies comparing different populations, cultures, and geographic regions; (2) studies comparing different individuals within a population; and, more recently, (3) intervention studies that attempt to alter dietary salt intake and assess the effects on BP.

A number of reports have compared salt intake and BP among different populations [6–16]. The majority of these studies found a positive correlation between sodium intake and the prevalence of high BP among various populations. Hypertension was found to be uncommon in populations with low dietary sodium intake. The amount of dietary sodium ranged from 1.5 mEq/day in the Yanomamo Indians of Brazil (with a negligible incidence of hypertension) to 425 mEq/day in northern Japanese (with a hypertension prevalence of 40%) [17]. These studies describe a relationship between dietary sodium intake and hypertension, but they are not specific about the amount of salt intake that may diminish the complications of hypertension. In extreme ranges of salt intake, most investigators observed differences in BP. However, whether limitations of salt intake within the range of the Western diet can affect BP is less certain.

Studies of within-population variation (i.e., a city or region with a diverse genetic composition) of the salt-BP relationship attempted to clarify the observations made in the interpopulation studies noted above. Elliott [18] presented an overview analysis of 14 studies that compared 24-hour urinary sodium excretion (as an acceptable measure of sodium intake) and BP. Included were studies within populations that examined the relationship of sodium intake to both systolic blood pressure (SBP) and diastolic blood pressure (DBP). The analysis included more than 12,000 adults. Significant positive relations were reported for BP and urinary sodium excretion. For men and women combined, regression estimates showed SBP decreased by 3.7 mm Hg and DBP decreased by 2.0 mm Hg, when 24-hour urinary sodium excretion was lowered by 100 mmol. Similar results were seen in the INTERSALT study, an international cooperative study on electrolytes and other factors related to BP involving 10,079 people [19]. The study reported a significant positive correlation between 24-hour urinary sodium excretion and SBP. The salt-BP relationship became stronger with increasing age.

It has been more difficult to demonstrate intrapopulation differences in dietary sodium and BP among children. Grobbee and Bak [20] reviewed sodium intake and BP in children and found variable results (Table 5.2). The studies reviewed documented sodium intake based on patient and family reporting and quantification of urinary sodium excretion. Their analysis demonstrates a weak correlation between salt intake and BP in children. This relationship is more pronounced in older individuals and in hypertensive individuals. A weakness of the studies is the difficulty in documenting sodium intake based on patient or family reporting. Therefore, the data from intrapopulation studies of sodium intake in children provide only weak evidence for a role for dietary salt restriction.

A more useful way to examine the relationship of salt intake and BP is through intervention studies that attempt to modify the dietary sodium content of individuals and assess the response of BP. Adult intervention studies confirm that in both across-population (studies comparing populations from unique geographic and cultural regions) and within-population (studies comparing individuals within a defined geographic region) studies, sodium restriction reduces BP. However, the response is greater in both subjects with higher initial BPs and in older adults [4, 23]. Table 5.3 summarizes intervention studies of sodium restriction in pediatric populations. The majority of these studies show no significant BP response to salt restriction. A major pitfall of the pediatric studies is the relatively short time periods for dietary salt restriction, most ranging from 4 to 6 weeks. An exception is the study by Hofman [24], which followed 245 infants through the first year of life and found a significant, albeit small (2.1 mm Hg lower in the low sodium group), effect. Studies have not shown whether adult hypertension is, in part, related to a cumulative effect of salt ingestion over

TABLE 5.2
A Summary of Findings from Observational Studies on Sodium Intake and Blood Pressure in Children

Studies	Year	N	Age (Yrs)
Positive studies*			
Calabrese and Tuthill	1977	606	10
Cooper et al	1980	73	11–14
Hofman and Valkenburg	1980	348	8–12
Watson et al	1980	662	?
Persson	1984	233	8
Negative studies*			
Armstrong et al	1982	635	12–14
Cooper et al	1983	241	12
Connor et al	1984	115	10
Persson	1984	238	4
Persson	1984	267	13
Robertson	1984	2,740	?
Jenner et al	1988	984	9
Geleijnse et al [21]	1990	233	5–17
Zhu et al [22]	1987	148	7–8

*"Positive" studies demonstrated a relationship between urinary sodium excretion and/or reported sodium intake with blood pressure. "Negative" studies demonstrated no such association.
Source: Modified from DE Grobbee, AAA Bak. Electrolyte Intake and Hypertension in Children. In R Rettig, D Ganten, FC Luft (eds), Salt and Hypertension: Dietary Minerals, Volume Homeostasis, and Cardiovascular Regulation. Berlin: Springer-Verlag, 1989;283.

TABLE 5.3
Summary of Salt Restriction Intervention Studies in Children and Adolescents

Reference	N	Age	Design	Result
Hofman [24]	476	0–25 wks	Double blind	↓SBP (2.1 mm Hg)
Gillum [25]	55	6–9 yrs	↓Na or low vs control	No response
Tucker [26]	216	4–5 yrs	↓Na or low vs regular	Significant decrease
Cooper [27]	124	adolescent	Crossover	No response
Grobbee [28]	40	18–28 yrs	Crossover	No response
Howe [29]	21	11–14 yrs	Crossover	No response
Miller [30]	149	School age	12-week Na restriction	No change in SBP or DPB in girls

a lifetime. It is possible that physiologic changes occur in childhood but do not manifest as hypertension until later years. If this premise is accepted, a consistent alteration of BP with salt intake in children may not be seen, yet salt restriction would remain an important intervention.

The lack of a reproducible response to salt restriction may be related to age, yet the small size of these studies does not adequately rule out variations among individuals within a population. The question of whether some individuals in a population are "salt-sensitive" has received much attention in recent years. Indeed, if such individuals are identified, they can be targeted for aggressive salt restriction efforts.

To understand the role of salt in hypertension, recognition of the role of sodium in the maintenance of systemic BP is important. Under physiologic conditions, to sustain an adequate intravascular volume, the kidneys maintain sodium balance via the renin-angiotensin–aldosterone system (see Figure 3.5, Chapter 3). The existence of salt-sensitive hypertension indicates that there must be individuals whose renal, neurologic, or hormonal regulation of BP and sodium balance is altered.

Laragh and Pickering [31] divide hypertension into two major types: *high plasma renin* ("dry vasoconstriction")—characterized by higher peripheral resistance, low plasma volume, reduced cardiac output, hemoconcentration, and postural hypotension; and *low plasma renin* ("wet vasoconstriction")—characterized by high plasma volume, high cardiac output, hemodilution, and high intravascular volume (Figure 5.1). Renovascular hypertension is an example of high plasma renin hypertension. Primary aldosteronism (e.g., Conn's disease) is an example of low-renin hypertension. Essential hypertension may fit into either of these categories, with various components of both high-renin and low-renin mechanisms contributing to hypertension. A patient's response to salt restriction may depend on whether vasoconstrictive or volume-mediated mechanisms predominate.

Salt-sensitive animal models have been described [32], with genetically transmitted salt sensitivity. Studies of the Dahl salt-sensitive rat suggest the presence of a hypertensionogenic substance in the circulation [33]. This substance has not been identified, but a number of characteristics of the Dahl salt-sensitive rat have been described that may help elucidate the mechanisms of salt sensitivity in humans [34] (Table 5.4).

Human studies also suggest that certain populations exhibit salt sensitivity. Factors other than age may contribute to the reductions in BP seen in patients following salt restriction. In contrast with Western populations, populations with low dietary salt consumption do not demonstrate age-related increases in BP [36]. Blacks demonstrate increased salt sensitivity when compared with whites at a similar age [37, 38]. Although the mechanism of salt sensitivity has not been completely elucidated, a number of characteristics are seen among people with an enhanced BP response to salt loading [32] (Table 5.5).

A model of salt-sensitive hypertension has been proposed [39]. In this model, increased dietary sodium intake, combined with the failure to adequately excrete a sodium load, stimulates the secretion of natriuretic factors. These natriuretic factors promote sodium excretion by

PATHOPHYSIOLOGIC DIFFERENCES

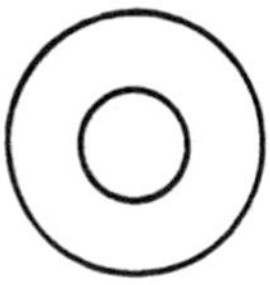

Arterioles

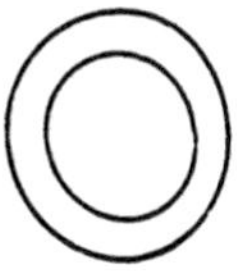

Higher	Peripheral resistance	High
High	Aldosterone	Low to High
Low	Plasma volume	High
Low	Cardiac output	High
High	Hematocrit	Low
High	Blood urea	Low
High	Blood viscosity	Low
Low	Tissue perfusion	High
Yes	Postural hypotension	No

CLINICAL EXAMPLES

High-renin essential hypertension
Renovascular and
malignant hypertension

Low-renin essential
hypertension
Primary aldosteronism

VASCULAR SEQUELAE

(+)	Stroke	(−)
(+)	Heart attack	(−)
(+)	Renal damage	(−)
(+)	Retinopathy-encephalopathy	(−)

TREATMENTS

(+)	Converting enzyme inhibitors	(−)
(+)	Beta blockers	(−)
(−)	Calcium channel blockers	(+)
(−)	Diuretics	(+)
(−)	Alpha blockers	(+)

FIGURE 5.1. Comparison of high-renin and low-renin forms of hypertension. (Reproduced with permission from JH Laragh, TG Pickering. Essential Hypertension. In BM Brenner, FC Rector [eds], The Kidney [4th ed]. Philadelphia: Saunders, 1991;1922.)

TABLE 5.4
Some Characteristics of the Dahl Salt-Sensitive Rat

Alterations of the autonomic nervous system with regard to vascular resistance
Decreased renal and plasma renin activity
Decreased renal Na,K-ATPase activity
Decreased urinary prostaglandin E_2 synthesis and excretion
Increased adrenal synthesis of 18-hydroxydeoxycorticosterone
Decreased plasma-aldosterone levels
Increased antidiuretic hormone release during high salt intake
Suppressed adrenal renin activity

Source: Modified with permission from DF Bohr, AF Dominiczak. Experimental hypertension. Hypertension 1991;17:39; and LK Dahl, G Leitl, M Heine. Influence of dietary potassium and sodium/potassium molar ratios on the development of salt hypertension. J Exp Med 1972;136:318.

TABLE 5.5
Characteristics of Salt-Sensitive Individuals

Enhanced blood pressure response to sodium depletion or repletion
Higher baseline blood pressure
Higher forearm vascular resistance, particularly with sodium loading
Suppressed renin release during sodium depletion
Reduced circulating aldosterone levels
A shift in the blood pressure–natriuresis relationship

---

inhibiting sodium reabsorption in renal tubular cells. These factors also inhibit sodium pumps in other cells, including vascular smooth muscle cells, causing intracellular sodium concentrations to increase. Increased intracellular sodium concentrations lead to increased intracellular calcium concentrations in the vascular smooth muscle cells, mediated by a Na-Ca exchange-transport system that attempts to pump out the extra sodium at the expense of increasing intracellular calcium. Increased intracellular calcium increases contractility and reactivity, thus manifesting as increased vascular tone and peripheral vascular resistance resulting in elevated BP. However, the following major questions remain unanswered about salt-mediated hypertension:

1. What is the nature of the defect(s) in renal sodium excretion?
2. What is the nature of the circulating natriuretic factors, the cellular potassium pump inhibitors, or both?
3. What amount of sodium intake is needed to cause hypertension in a given individual?

Until these areas can be further clarified, the identification of salt-sensitive individuals is based on trials of salt restriction.

With regard to question one, studies have identified increased red blood cell lithium-sodium countertransport in patients with essential hypertension [40]. Weder [41] showed that white males with essential hypertension had increased proximal renal tubular reabsorption of sodium, and that red cell lithium-sodium countertransport may be a marker of that tendency. Others have questioned whether lithium-sodium countertransport is the mechanism of increased intracellular sodium, or simply a marker of a tendency toward altered membrane sodium transport [42]. Other sodium transport mechanisms have been identified including sodium-potassium–ATPase [43]. However, there is no consensus regarding which of the transport mechanisms is altered in essential hypertension.

With regard to question two, Dahl demonstrated a hypertensiono-genic substance in the blood of salt-sensitive rats in parabiotic experiments [33]. Some human studies postulated a circulating inhibitor of sodium transport as the human analog of this substance. One possibility is that of circulating inhibitors of Na,K-ATPase. De Wardener [44] proposed the following possible mechanism: "normal plasma and hypothalamus contain volume-controlled Na,K-ATPase–inhibitory activity. The intensity of this activity in the plasma and hypothalamic extracts is raised in acquired and essential hypertension." While much remains to be explained, it appears that salt sensitivity is mediated by alterations in intracellular sodium transport mechanisms and their mediators, and that some of these alterations may be inherited.

With regard to question three, further clarification of the role of salt in hypertension may be found in studies that demonstrate the importance of the anion that accompanies sodium [45, 46]. In experiments comparing the effect of sodium chloride with sodium and other anions, as well as chloride and other cations, the development of increased BP was most consistent with high intakes of sodium chloride [46]. The mechanism for this dependence on sodium chloride is unclear but may be related to the influence of the anion on the distribution of sodium between the intracellular and extracellular compartments. Thus, it is more appropriate to refine question three above to include only sodium chloride.

From the above discussion, we see that among hypertensive individuals, there are some who respond to salt restriction as a means of lowering BP. Although the mechanisms of salt sensitivity continue to be elucidated, as yet there is no clinically useful way to choose which individuals will respond without a trial of salt restriction. Therefore, we recommend a trial of a low-salt diet in the initial therapy of essential hypertension. This may be difficult for younger children, particularly in families where high salt intake is the norm. Salt restriction may also potentiate the effects of antihypertensive medications, and consequently lower doses of medications may be needed in patients on low-salt diets.

However, it is also important to note that there are some populations in which salt restriction may be detrimental. In particular, those with excessive salt losses (urinary, sweat, etc.) may be more susceptible to some of the effects of salt restriction that have been identified, such as increased renin and norepinephrine levels [47].

What is a salt-restricted diet? The average American adult ingests approximately 200 mEq/day of sodium (43.5 mEq = 1 g). A reduction of sodium intake by one-half (to 100 mEq/day) in adults reduces SBP and DBP by 5 and 6 mm Hg, respectively [17]. For younger children, parents must be willing to carefully monitor their children's diets, and interventions may be most effective if salt intake is also limited for the household. For adolescents, compliance is particularly difficult, with many meals eaten outside of the home. School-based programs have met with mixed results.

Potassium Supplementation

Studies in both animals [35, 48] and humans [4, 21, 28, 49, 50] have described an antihypertensive effect of potassium supplementation. This effect is small and not consistently observed. Low-sodium diets are necessarily higher in potassium content, and the contribution of potassium may be underestimated. A possible mechanism for the antihypertensive effect of potassium involves a potassium-induced natriuresis. While increased dietary potassium may increase aldosterone secretion and thereby blunt any BP-lowering effect of a potassium-induced natriuresis, the relationship between the intracellular transport of both sodium and potassium remains unclear. Investigators have observed sustained BP reduction in potassium-supplemented diets. Potassium may also affect the central or autonomic nervous system regulation of BP by (1) increasing the sensitivity of the baroreceptor response, (2) preventing the increase of catecholamines seen in sodium restriction [17], or (3) acting through a mechanism that has not yet been identified. At present, there are no convincing studies in children recommending dietary potassium supplementation as a therapy for hypertension.

Calcium Supplementation

Earlier in this chapter, models of essential hypertension in which sodium was responsible for modifying BP were reviewed. In those models, increased intracellular calcium, which results in increased vascular tone, is the endpoint that leads to increased BP [51]. Therefore, one would expect that dietary calcium impacts control of BP much like sodium. What is not intuitively clear is whether calcium restriction or calcium supplementation lowers BP.

TABLE 5.6
Mechanisms of Blood Pressure Modification by Intracellular Calcium

---

Smooth muscle contraction (particularly vascular)
Cardiac contractility
Stimulus-secretion coupling of endocrine and neuroendocrine responses
    Renin-aldosterone system
    Parathyroid hormone and vitamin D
    Neurotransmitter release (epinephrine, norepinephrine)
Intrinsic renal function
    Renal tubular sodium and calcium transport
    Renin secretion

Although it is widely believed that increased intracellular calcium is necessary for hypertension to develop, there are a variety of mechanisms through which intracellular calcium may exert its effect (Table 5.6). Clinical studies have shown a variety of conflicting responses to increased dietary calcium—with many showing a decrease in BP with calcium supplementation [52–61] and others showing no BP response to calcium supplementation [62–66]. The variety of responses may represent a small effect, or more likely, suggest that a subset of both hypertensive and normotensive populations respond to calcium supplementation, and the effect is diminished when nonresponders are included in the studies.

Paradoxically, essential hypertension is related to increased intracellular calcium concentrations, although a majority of the studies show that BP decreases in response to increased dietary calcium. A model to explain this apparent incongruity has been proposed by Resnick [54] (Figure 5.2). In this model, essential hypertension falls between two parameters. In both, increased intracellular calcium is responsible for increasing BP possibly through one or more of the mechanisms listed in Table 5.6.

The first category of essential hypertension in Figure 5.2 involves low-renin hypertension (see Figure 5.1), in which serum-ionized calcium levels are low and intracellular calcium concentration is elevated. Resnick [54] refers to this as a type I defect. It is characterized by a cell membrane–mediated altered distribution between intracellular and extracellular calcium pools. This form of hypertension would more likely respond to calcium supplementation and calcium channel blockade. As discussed in the section on salt sensitivity, this category of patients may have a sodium transport–mediated effect on calcium distribution and therefore respond to salt restriction by altering the relative concentrations of intra- and extracellular calcium. The second category (type II defect) is characterized by high renin. With this defect, the extracellular calcium pool (measured as ionized calcium) is normal or increased. The high cytosolic concentration of calcium is based on a defect in intracellular distribution, perhaps among

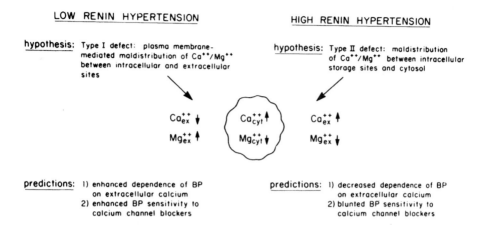

LOW RENIN HYPERTENSION

hypothesis: Type I defect: plasma membrane-mediated maldistribution of Ca^{++}/Mg^{++} between intracellular and extracellular sites

HIGH RENIN HYPERTENSION

hypothesis: Type II defect: maldistribution of Ca^{++}/Mg^{++} between intracellular storage sites and cytosol

$Ca_{ex}^{++} \downarrow$

$Mg_{ex}^{++} \uparrow$

$Ca_{cyt}^{++} \uparrow$

$Mg_{cyt}^{++} \downarrow$

$Ca_{ex}^{++} \uparrow$

$Mg_{ex}^{++} \downarrow$

predictions: 1) enhanced dependence of BP on extracellular calcium
2) enhanced BP sensitivity to calcium channel blockers

predictions: 1) decreased dependence of BP on extracellular calcium
2) blunted BP sensitivity to calcium channel blockers

FIGURE 5.2. Spectrum of essential hypertension. (Reproduced with permission from LM Resnick. Uniformity and diversity of calcium metabolism in hypertension. A conceptual framework. Am J Med 1987;82(Suppl 1B):20.)

cytosol and organelles such as mitochondria, endoplasmic reticulum, or other modulators of cellular homeostasis. Because this type of defect is not dependent on fluxes of calcium across the cell membrane, patients with this form of hypertension are less likely to respond to calcium supplementation, calcium channel blockers, and sodium restriction. Despite continued progress in elucidating the role of dietary calcium in hypertension, there is no clinically reproducible way to identify those patients who might respond to calcium supplementation. As research progresses in basic science (e.g., ATP-dependent, transmembrane calcium transport, intracellular calcium–binding capacity, and the role of sodium transport mechanisms) and clinical medicine (e.g., characterization of salt- and calcium-sensitive individuals based on sodium-renin profiling, ionized calcium levels, renal calcium excretion, plasma parathyroid hormone levels, etc.) recommendations on dietary modifications in hypertension should be forthcoming.

Magnesium Supplementation

Magnesium is the principal intracellular divalent cation. It is involved in the physiology of sodium, potassium, and calcium and is essential for many cellular processes. For example, Na,K-ATPase, calcium-dependent potassium channels, Ca-ATPase, and a variety of other transport mechanisms are influenced by intracellular magnesium concentrations [67]. Clinically, the hypotensive effect of magnesium in pre-eclampsia and in malignant hypertension suggests a role for magnesium supplementation in

TABLE 5.7
Characteristics of Obesity-Associated Hypertension

Increased activity of the sympathetic nervous system
Sodium retention or decreased sodium excretion
Increased cardiac output
Increased intravascular volume
Myocardial hypertrophy
Upper body fat distribution
Hyperinsulinemia/insulin resistance

---

essential hypertension. Some studies have shown a limited hypotensive response to magnesium, primarily in patients in a relatively potassium-depleted state [67–69], but results are insufficient to recommend magnesium supplementation as a treatment for hypertension. It has been suggested [54] that decreased intracellular magnesium concentrations, in conjunction with increased intracellular calcium concentrations, may be a central factor in the development of essential hypertension, but the precise mechanisms have not been elucidated.

Weight Loss

Obesity and hypertension are strongly correlated (see Chapter 7). While the mechanisms of hypertension-associated obesity are incompletely understood, the efficacy of weight loss as a treatment for hypertension is clear. The relationship of obesity to hypertension has been well described in children and adolescents [70–78]. In attempting to understand the mechanisms of obesity-associated hypertension, researchers have made several observations about what may be responsible for the increase in BP (Table 5.7). The activity of the sympathetic nervous system is increased in obese hypertensive patients [79]. Weight loss, as well as diets low in carbohydrates and fats, reduce sympathetic activity in association with reduction of BP [80]. Rocchini [73] demonstrated that the hypotensive response of weight loss in adolescents is heightened by sodium restriction, and it has been postulated that obese individuals are in a salt-retaining state, with hyperinsulinemia or increased sympathetic activity as the cause [81]. In addition to increased sympathetic activity and sodium retention, obesity has been associated with increased cardiac output and intravascular volume [82–84], and with myocardial hypertrophy that is independent of the left ventricular hypertrophy seen in hypertension alone [82]. The distribution of body fat in obesity also appears to play a role in the development of hypertension. In particular, an upper body fat distribution with a higher waist-to-hip ratio is associated with hypertension [85, 86].

Can a single mechanism account for the above observations? Obese patients are in either a hyperinsulinemic or insulin-resistant state, or both [73, 76, 87–90]. A hyperinsulinemic state may explain some of the characteristics of obese hypertensive patients. Elevated insulin levels are implicated in the increased sympathetic activity observed in obese hypertensive patients [91]. Insulin has an antinatriuretic effect on the kidney [75] and may be, in part, responsible for the sodium-sensitive nature of hypertension in many obese individuals. Upper body obesity appears to correlate more strongly with hyperinsulinemia than lower body obesity [92].

Based on these observations, Landsberg [93] suggested that a major component of obesity-associated hypertension involves a state of hyperinsulinemia and insulin resistance (Figure 5.3). In patients ingesting excess calories, insulin secretion is stimulated, resulting in obesity and the subsequent development of insulin resistance. This creates a cycle of increasing insulin secretion, adipocyte hypertrophy, obesity, and insulin resistance. In this state, while the adipocytes remain resistant to the effects of insulin, other body tissues retain their responsiveness to insulin and maintain a response that leads to hypertension. In particular, increased sympathetic nervous system activity, renal salt retention, increased intravascular volume, and vasoconstriction may contribute to the elevated BP.

Studies have failed to show a sustained hypertensive response to chronic insulin infusion in obese, insulin-resistant dogs [94], suggesting that other mechanisms are involved. While Landsberg's hypothesis attempts to explain only part of the complex mechanisms of BP control, it provides a rationale for the use of diet and weight loss as treatments of hypertension.

Obesity is a serious problem among adolescents in Western society. Many children and adolescents evaluated for hypertension are obese. Caloric restriction, weight loss, and exercise independently reduce BP [81, 95]. Sodium restriction may be particularly important in obese individuals. In patients requiring medication, control of obesity may reduce the dosage or number of medications required to maintain BP control.

Exercise

The role of exercise and hypertension, with particular emphasis on types of exercise appropriate for patients with hypertension, is discussed in Chapter 7.

Cardiovascular Risk Factor Modification

While the reduction of BP is important in preventing or delaying cardiovascular morbidity and mortality, it is only part of a strategy. Efforts to reduce cardiovascular disease and stroke in adulthood must also include attention

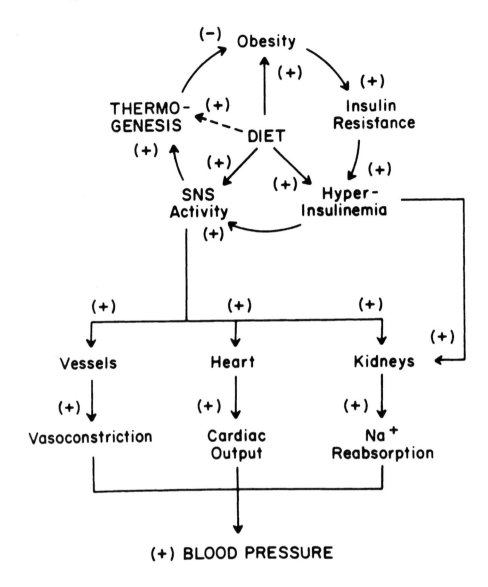

FIGURE 5.3. Relationship between hyperinsulinemia, insulin resistance, and hypertension. (Reproduced with permission from L Landsberg. Diet, obesity, and hypertension: a hypothesis involving insulin. The sympathetic nervous system, and adaptive thermogenesis. Q J Med 1986;236:1085. By permission of Oxford University Press.)

to smoking, hypercholesterolemia or hyperlipidemia, stressful lifestyles, and physical inactivity [96].

Smoking remains a serious health risk among adolescents. In the United States, approximately 30% of adolescents report smoking at least once monthly [97]; in England, an estimated 500,000 smokers age 11–15 are reported [98]. Although the numbers of adolescent smokers are declining, tobacco companies target children and adolescents in their advertising campaigns. Due to social and peer pressure, family influences, and lack of education regarding the risks of smoking, cigarettes will continue to be a major health problem for the foreseeable future. Ongoing efforts to prevent smoking in children must continue, and patients with hypertension must be made aware of their increased risk.

Much controversy exists over the role of childhood and adolescent hypercholesterolemia and hyperlipidemia in the development of adult cardiovascular disease. Current recommendations regarding when and whom to test vary, ranging from universal testing of all children over the age of 2, to no testing at all [99]. The National Cholesterol Education Program of the National Heart, Lung, and Blood Institute has published recommendations regarding screening and treatment of hypercholesterolemia in children and adolescents [100]. Because of the added risk of hypercholesterolemia in hypertensive individuals, fasting lipid profiles (total cholesterol, high-density lipoprotein and low-density lipoprotein cholesterol, triglycerides) should be obtained in hypertensive children and adolescents. Identification of familial lipid disorders and of children with abnormal lipid profiles will facilitate treatment and should continue in conjunction with antihypertensive therapy.

Summary

Nonpharmacologic therapy is an important first step in the treatment of hypertension in children and adolescents, as well as an adjunct to pharmacologic therapy. Sodium restriction, weight loss, and exercise are effective therapies. For patients with borderline hypertension, we recommend a trial of dietary salt and calorie restriction under the supervision of a dietician. We also encourage a regular exercise program. A 6-month period is usually sufficient to determine whether these interventions will be effective. We stress to patients that compliance with nonpharmacologic measures may prevent or delay the need for a lifetime of medication. As those who have tried to use nonpharmacologic therapies can attest, compliance with dietary and exercise recommendations is often poor. Viskoper has suggested several ways to improve patient compliance in these therapies [101]. These suggestions are summarized in Table 5.8. Understanding of the role of potassium, calcium, magnesium, and other (unidentified) factors continues to develop.

TABLE 5.8
Suggestions for Improving Compliance with Nonpharmacologic Blood Pressure
Reduction Therapies

1. Provide age-specific information on the health hazards of hypertension and other risk factors for cardiovascular disease.
2. Develop specific written short- and long-term treatment goals to be given to the patient.
3. Be encouraging: Positive reinforcement is more effective than negative reinforcement.
4. Try to discover motivational factors unique to each patient (i.e., improved physical appearance, improved athletic performance, improved self-esteem).
5. Identify specific problem areas with compliance rather than declare a patient to be "noncompliant."
6. Involve the patient's family: It is difficult to be the only one in a household with dietary restrictions.

References

1. Ambard L, Beaujard E. Causes de l'hypertension arterielle. Arch Gen Med 1904;1:520.
2. Chockalingham A, Abbott D, Bass M, et al. Recommendations of the Canadian consensus on nonpharmacological approaches to the management of high BP. Can Med Assoc J 1990;142:1397.
3. Jung FF, Ingelfinger JR. Hypertension in childhood and adolescence. Pediatr Rev 1993;14:169.
4. Langford HG. Nonpharmacological therapy of hypertension: commentary on diet and BP. Hypertension 1989;13(Suppl I):98.
5. Elmer PJ, Grimm RH, Flack J, Laing B. Dietary sodium reduction for hypertension prevention and treatment. Hypertension 1991;17:182.
6. Dahl LK. Possible Role of Salt Intake in the Development of Essential Hypertension. In P Cottier, KD Bock (eds), Essential Hypertension—An International Symposium. Berlin: Springer-Verlag, 1960;53.
7. Burns-Cox CJ, Maclean JD. Splenomegaly and blood pressure in an Orang Asli community in West Malaysia. Am Heart J 1970;80:718.
8. Cruz-Coke R, Etcheverry R, Nagel R. Influence of migration on blood pressure of Easter Islanders. Lancet 1964;1:697.
9. Lowenstein FW. Blood pressure in relation to age and sex in the tropics and subtropics: a review of the literature and an investigation in two tribes of Brazil Indians. Lancet 1961;1:389.
10. Maddocks I. Blood pressures in Melanesians. Med J Aust 1967;1:1123.
11. Page LB. Epidemiologic evidence on the etiology of human hypertension and its possible prevention. Am Heart J 1976;91:527.
12. Page LB, Danion A, Moellering RC. Antecedents to cardiovascular disease in six Solomon Islands societies. Circulation 1974;49:1132.

13. Prior AM, Evans JG, Harvey HBP. Sodium intake and blood pressure in two Polynesian populations. N Engl J Med 1968;279:515.

14. Tsugane S, Kitagawa Y, Kondo H. Ethnic differences in blood pressure level between Japanese school children in Bolivia and native Bolivians. Int J Epidemiol 1989;18:100.

15. Gleibermann L. Blood pressure and dietary salt in human populations. Ecol Food Nutri 1973;2:143.

16. Froment A, Milon H, Gravier C. Relation entre consommation sodee et hypertension arterielle. Rev Epidemiol Sante Publique 1979;27:437.

17. McMahon FG. Hypertension: The Once-A-Day Era (3rd ed). Mount Kisco, NY: Futura, 1990.

18. Elliott P. Observational studies of salt and blood pressure. Hypertension 1991;17:I3.

19. Stamler J, Rose G, Elliott P, et al. Findings of the International Cooperative INTERSALT study. Hypertension 1991;17:9.

20. Grobbee DE, Bak AAA. Electrolyte Intake and Hypertension in Children. In R Rettig, D Ganten, FC Luft (eds), Salt and Hypertension: Dietary Minerals, Volume Homeostasis, and Cardiovascular Regulation. Berlin: Springer-Verlag, 1989;283.

21. Geleijnse JM, Grobbee DE, Hofman A. Sodium and potassium intake and blood pressure change in childhood. Br Med J 1990;300:899.

22. Zhu K, He S, Pan X, et al. The relation of urinary cations to blood pressure in boys aged seven to eight years. Am J Epidemiol 1987;126:658.

23. Cutler JA, Follman D, Elliott P, Suh I. An overview of randomized trials of sodium reduction and blood pressure. Hypertension 1991;17:I27.

24. Hofman A, Hazebroek A, Valkenburg HA. A randomized trial of sodium intake and blood pressure in newborn infants. JAMA 1983;250:370.

25. Gillum RF, Elmer PJ, Prineas RJ. Changing sodium intake in children: the Minneapolis Children's Blood Pressure study. Hypertension 1981;3:698.

26. Tucker DT, Smothers M, Lewis C, Feldman H. Effects of decreased dietary salt intake on blood pressure in preschool children. J Natl Med Assoc 1983;81: 299.

27. Cooper R, Van Horn L, Liu K, et al. A randomized trial on the effect of decreased dietary sodium intake on blood pressure in adolescents. J Hypertens 1984;2:361.

28. Grobbee DE, Hofman A, Roelandt JT, et al. Sodium restriction and potassium supplementation in young people with mildly elevated blood pressure. J Hypertens 1987;5:115.

29. Howe PRC, Cobiac L, Smith RM. Lack of effect of short-term changes in sodium intake on blood pressure in adolescent schoolchildren. J Hypertens 1991;9:181.

30. Miller JZ, Weinberger MH, Daugherty SA, et al. Blood pressure response to dietary sodium restriction in normotensive children. Am J Clin Nutr 1988;47:113.

31. Laragh JH, Pickering TG. Essential Hypertension. In BM Brenner, FC Rector (eds), The Kidney (4th ed). Philadelphia: Saunders, 1991;1909.

32. Sullivan JM. Salt sensitivity: definition, conception, methodology, and long-term issues. Hypertension 1991;17:61.
33. Dahl LK, Knudson KD, Iwai J. Humoral transmission of hypertension: evidence from parabiosis. Circ Res 1969;25(Suppl I);21.
34. Bohr DF, Dominiczak AF. Experimental hypertension. Hypertension 1991;17:39.
35. Tobian L. Salt and hypertension: lessons from animal models that relate to human hypertension. Hypertension 1991;17:52.
36. Weinberger MH, Fineberg NS. Sodium and volume sensitivity of blood pressure. Age and pressure change over time. Hypertension 1991;18:67.
37. Luft FC, Miller JZ, Grim CE, et al. Salt sensitivity and resistance of blood pressure: age and race as factors in physiological responses. Hypertension 1991;17:102.
38. Harshfield GA, Alpert BS, Pulliam DA, et al. Sodium excretion and racial differences in ambulatory blood pressure patterns. Hypertension 1991;18:813.
39. Blaustein MP, Hamlyn JM. Sodium transport inhibition, cell calcium, and hypertension: the natriuretic hormone/Na-Ca exchange/hypertension hypothesis. Am J Med 1984;5:45.
40. Canessa M, Adragna N, Solomon HS, et al. Increased sodium-lithium countertransport in red cells of patients with essential hypertension. N Engl J Med 1980;302:772.
41. Weder AB. Membrane sodium transport and salt sensitivity of blood pressure. Hypertension 1991;17:I74.
42. Hilton PJ. Cellular sodium transport in essential hypertension. N Engl J Med 1986;314: 222.
43. Trevisan M, Krogh V, Dorn J, DeSanto NG. Blood pressure and intracellular ion transport in childhood. Semin Nephrol 1989;9:253.
44. De Wardener HE. Kidney, salt intake, and Na,K-ATPase inhibitors in hypertension. Hypertension 1991;17:830.
45. Hanna JD, Chan J. Hypertension and the kidney. J Pediatr 1991;118:327.
46. Boegehold MA, Kotchen TA. Importance of dietary chloride for salt sensitivity of blood pressure. Hypertension 1991;17:158.
47. Dimsdale JE, Ziegler M, Mills P, Berry C. Prediction of salt sensitivity. Am J Hypertens 1990;3:429.
48. Dahl LK, Leitl G, Heine M. Influence of dietary potassium and sodium/potassium molar ratios on the development of salt hypertension. J Exp Med 1972;136:318.
49. Langford HG, Watson RL. Electrolytes and Hypertension. In O Paul (ed), Epidemiology and Control of Hypertension. Chicago: Year Book, 1975;103.
50. Watson RL, Langford HG, Abernethy J, et al. Urinary electrolytes, body weight, and blood pressure. Hypertension 1980;2:93.
51. Grobbee DE, Waal-Manning HJ. The role of calcium supplementation in the treatment of hypertension: current evidence. Drugs 1990;39:7.
52. Belizan JM, Villar J, Pineda O. Reduction of blood pressure with calcium in young adults. JAMA 1983;249:1161.

53. Lyle RM, Melby CL, Hyner GC, et al. Blood pressure and metabolic effects of calcium supplementation in normotensive white and black men. JAMA 1987;257:1771.
54. Resnick LM. The Role of Dietary Calcium and Magnesium in the Therapy of Hypertension. In JH Laragh and BM Brenner (eds), Hypertension: Pathophysiology, Diagnosis, and Management. New York: Raven, 1990;2037.
55. Johnson NE, Smith EL, Freudenheim JL. Effects on blood pressure of calcium supplementation of women. Am J Clin Nutr 1985;42:12.
56. McCarron DA. A consensus approach to electrolytes and blood pressure: could we all be right? Hypertension 1991;17:170.
57. Zemel MB, Gualdoni SM, Sowers JR. Reduction in total and extracellular water associated with calcium-induced natriuresis and the antihypertensive effect of calcium in blacks. Am J Hypertens 1988;1:70.
58. Grobbee DE, Hofman A. Effect of calcium supplementation on diastolic blood pressure in young people with mild hypertension. Lancet 1986;2:703.
59. Tabuchi Y, Ogihara T, Hashizume K, et al. Hypertensive effect of long-term oral calcium supplementation in elderly patients with essential hypertension. J Clin Hypertens 1986;3:254.
60. Lasiridis AN, Zanaieri KI, Kaisis CN, et al. Oral calcium supplementation promotes renal sodium excretion in essential hypertension. J Hypertens 1987;5(Suppl 5):307.
61. Repke JT, Villar J, Anderson C, et al. Biochemical changes associated with blood pressure reduction induced by calcium supplementation during pregnancy. Am J Obstet Gynecol 1989;160:684.
62. Thomsen K, Nilas L, Christiansen C. Dietary calcium intake and blood pressure in normotensive subjects. Acta Med Scand 1987;222:51.
63. Meese RB, Gonzales DG, Casparian JM, et al. The inconsistent effects of calcium supplements upon blood pressure in primary hypertension. Am J Med Sci 1987;254:219.
64. Strazullo P, Siani A, Gugliemi S. Controlled trial of long-term oral calcium supplementation in essential hypertension. Hypertension 1986;8:1084.
65. Nowson C, Morgan T. Effect of calcium carbonate on blood pressure. J Hypertens 1986;4(Suppl 6):673.
66. Zoccali C, Mallamaci F, Delfino D. Does calcium have a dual effect on arterial pressure? Response to 1,25 dihydroxyvitamin D_3 and calcium supplements in essential hypertension. J Hypertens 1987;5(Suppl 5):267.
67. Motoyama T, Sano H, Fukuzuki H. Oral magnesium supplementation in patients with essential hypertension. Hypertension 1989;13:227.
68. Reyes AJ, Leary WP, Acosta-Barrios TN, Davis WH. Magnesium supplementation in hypertension treated with hydrochlorothiazide. Current Therapy 1984;36:322.
69. Saito K, Hattori K, Omatsu T. Effects of oral magnesium on blood pressure and red cell sodium transport in patients receiving long-term thiazide diuretics for hypertension. Am J Hypertens 1988;1:71.
70. Clarke WR, Woolson RF, Lauer RM. Changes in ponderosity and blood pressure in childhood: The Muscatine study. Am J Epidemiol 1986;124:195.

71. Staessen J, Fagard R, Amery A. Obesity and hypertension. Acta Cardiol 1988;(Suppl) 29:37.
72. Thomas PW, Peters TJ, Golding J, Haslum MN. Height, weight, and blood pressure in ten-year-old children. Hum Biol 1989;61:213.
73. Rocchini AP. Cardiovascular regulation in obesity-induced hypertension. Hypertension 1992;19(Suppl I):I56.
74. Berenson GS, Webber LS, Srinivasan SR. Pathogenesis of hypertension in black and white children. Clin Cardiol 1989;12(Suppl 4):3.
75. Gupta AK, Clark RV, Kirchner KA. Effects of insulin on renal sodium excretion. Hypertension 1992;19(Suppl I):I78.
76. Kanai H, Matsuzawa Y, Tokunaga K, et al. Hypertension in obese children: fasting serum insulin levels are closely correlated with blood pressure. Int J Obes 1990;14:1047.
77. Lauer RM, Burns TL, Clarke WR, Mahoney LT. Childhood predictors of future blood pressure. Hypertension 1991;18(Suppl 3):74.
78. Gilbert TJ, Percy CA, Sugarman JR, et al. Obesity among Navajo adolescents: relationship to dietary intake and blood pressure. Am J Dis Child 1992;146:289.
79. Tuck ML. Obesity, the sympathetic nervous system, and essential hypertension. Hypertension 1992;19(Suppl I):67.
80. Jung RT, Shetty PS, Barrand M, et al. Role of catecholamines in hypotensive response to dieting. Br Med J 1979;1:12.
81. Krieger DR, Landsberg L. Obesity and Hypertension. In JH Laragh, BM Brenner (eds), Hypertension: Pathophysiology, Diagnosis, and Management. New York: Raven, 1990;1741.
82. Messerli FH, Sundgaard-Riise K, Reisin E, et al. Disparate cardiovascular effects of obesity and arterial hypertension. Am J Med 1983;74:808.
83. Mujais SK, Tarazi RC, Dustin HP, et al. Hypertension in obese patients: hemodynamic and volume studies. Hypertension 1982;4:84.
84. Raison HJ, Achimastos A, Bouthier J, et al. Intravascular volume, extracellular fluid volume, and total body water in obese and non-obese hypertensive patients. Am J Cardiol 1983;51:165.
85. Krotkiewski M, Bjorntorp P, Sjostrom L, Smith U. Impact of obesity on metabolism in men and women: importance of regional adipose tissue distribution. J Clin Invest 1983;72:1150.
86. Williams PT, Fortmann SP, Terry RB, et al. Associations of dietary fat, regional adiposity, and blood pressure in men. JAMA 1987;257:3251.
87. Ferrannini E, Buzzigoli G, Bonadonna R. Insulin resistance in essential hypertension. N Engl J Med 1987;317:350.
88. Lucas CP, Estigarribia JA, Darga LL, Reaven GM. Insulin and blood pressure in obesity. Hypertension 1985;7:702.
89. Manicardi V, Camellini L, Bellodi G, et al. Evidence for an association of high blood pressure and hyperinsulinemia in obese man. J Clin Endocrinol Metab 1986;62:1302.
90. Modan M, Halkin H, Almog S. Hyperinsulinemia: a link between hypertension, obesity, and glucose intolerance. J Clin Invest 1985;75:809.

The target BP should be under the ninety-fifth percentile for sex and age. The therapeutic approach in chronic renal failure is different than that of essential hypertension. In chronic renal failure, the therapy is directed at reducing volume expansion, sodium retention, and decreasing peripheral vascular resistance, which is secondary to vasoactive factors (such as nitric oxide) or changes in intrarenal hormone production (prostaglandins), the renin-angiotensin–aldosterone system, or the sympathetic nervous system. Figure 6.6 is an approach to treatment in patients with chronic kidney failure. Unless an emergent problem supervenes, it is important to wait several days after making dosage adjustments or adding new agents to assess the impact of BP control [80].

Diuretics are effective first-line therapy for hypertension in patients with sodium and water retention and a GFR above 10–15 ml/minute/1.73 m^2 (see Figure 6.6). With a GFR below 30–40 ml/minute/1.73 m^2, thiazide diuretics (hydrochlorothiazide, chlorothiazide, and metolazone) lose their ability to increase sodium delivery to the distal nephron and increase the loss of free water. The dosage modifications in renal failure are shown in Table 6.31.

In patients with decreased renal function (GFR <30–40 ml/minute/1.73 m^2), loop diuretics are more effective than thiazide diuretics. Potassium-sparing diuretics (spironolactone, triamterene, and amiloride) should be used with extreme caution in patients with renal failure.

Because of the high percentage of children with reactive airway disease who participate in athletics, beta-adrenergic blocking agents should be used with caution. The exception is labetalol with alpha-adrenergic antagonism in addition to beta-antagonism (about 1/10 of beta blockers), which is very effective in children with chronic renal failure.

Vasodilators in chronic renal failure are used primarily in the treatment of hypertensive urgencies and emergencies. Minoxidil is a potent vasodilator, but its use is limited because of sodium and fluid retention, incidence of pericardial effusions and congestive heart failure, and hypertrichosis (see Figure 6.6).

Despite the large number of different classes of antihypertensive agents, angiotensin-converting enzyme (ACE) inhibitors delay the rate of progression of renal failure. The use of ACE inhibitors in patients with moderate renal insufficiency (GFR <40–50 ml/minute/1.73 m^2) is problematic because while they delay progressive kidney injury and control hypertension, they may also compromise renal function, increase proteinuria, and cause hyperkalemia.

Calcium channel blockers are excellent first-line antihypertensive therapy and are not contraindicted in patients with renovascular hypertension secondary to bilateral renal artery stenosis.

The management of a child with chronic renal failure before the initiation of dialysis or transplantation (renal replacement therapy) is different from that of children without renal disease. In such cases, inadequate control

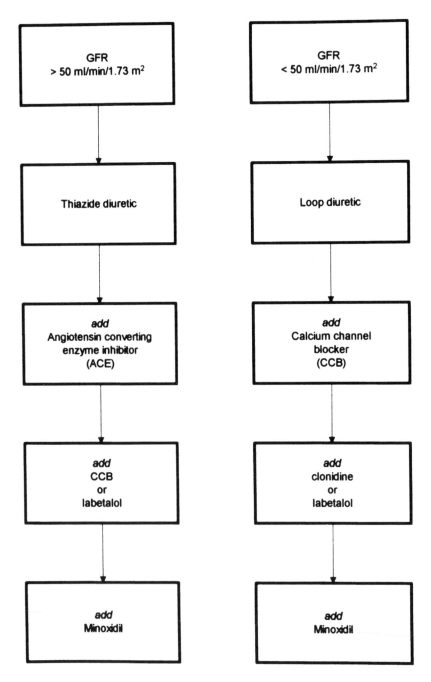

FIGURE 6.6. Suggested treatment approach for children with chronic renal insufficiency. (Reproduced with permission from LG Feld, E Lieberman, SA Mendoza, JE Springate. Management of hypertension in the child with chronic renal failure. J Pediatr 1996;129[Suppl]:S18.)

91. Landsberg L, Young JB. Insulin-mediated glucose metabolism in the relationship between dietary intake and sympathetic nervous system activity. Int J Obes 1985;9:63.

92. Kissebah AH, Vydelingum N, Murray R, et. al. Relation of body fat distribution to metabolic complications of obesity. J Clin Endocrinol Metab 1982;54:254.

93. Landsberg L. Hyperinsulinemia: possible role in obesity-induced hypertension. Hypertension 1992;19(Suppl I):61.

94. Hall JE, Brands MW, Hildebrandt DA, Mizelle HL. Obesity-associated hypertension: hyperinsulinemia and renal mechanisms. Hypertension 1992;19(Suppl I):45.

95. Fagard R, Bielen E, Hespel P, et al. Physical Exercise in Hypertension. In JH Laragh, BM Brenner (eds), Hypertension: Pathophysiology, Diagnosis, and Management. New York: Raven, 1990;1985.

96. Havas S, Wozenski S, Deprez R, et al. Report of the New England Task Force on Reducing Heart Disease and Stroke Risk. Public Health Rep 1989;104:134.

97. LaGreca AM, Fisher EB. Adolescent smoking. Pediatr Ann 1992;21:241.

98. Holland WW, Fitzsimons B. Smoking in children. Arch Dis Child 1991;66:1269.

99. Hoekelman RA. A pediatrician's view: cholesterol mania. Pediatr Ann 1992;21:215.

100. National Cholesterol Education Program. Report of the Expert Panel on Blood Cholesterol Levels in Children and Adolescents. Pediatrics 1992;89(Suppl):525.

101. Viskoper JR. Manual of Nonpharmcological Control of Hypertension. New York: Springer-Verlag, 1990;76.

CHAPTER 6

Pharmacologic Therapy of Hypertension

Leonard G. Feld and Wayne R. Waz

With our increasing understanding of the mechanisms that control blood pressure (BP), our ability to influence the development and maintenance of hypertension continues to improve. Current pharmacotherapy permits manipulation of the following:

Hormonal control of BP

Vascular control of BP

Cardiac control of BP

Volume-mediated control of BP

Central nervous system (CNS) control of BP

While some specific indications for particular classes of medications exist (e.g., angiotensin-converting enzyme inhibitors for high-renin hypertension), in the majority of cases there are multiple causes of elevated BP. Medication should therefore be chosen based on the need to both maximize reduction in BP and minimize side effects. Inasmuch as the ultimate goal of antihypertensive therapy is to prevent adverse cardiovascular events (i.e., stroke and myocardial infarction) and end-organ damage (i.e., retinopathy and nephropathy), medications should be evaluated in terms of their effect on myocardial size and function, possible metabolic derangements (e.g., lipid or blood glucose profiles), and side effects that cause patients to discontinue their use. This chapter reviews the major classes of antihypertensive drugs, with attention focused on medications commonly used in children and adolescents. Other, more comprehensive reviews have been published [1, 2].

Angiotensin-Converting Enzyme Inhibitors

Angiotensin-converting enzyme (ACE) inhibitors affect BP by blocking the conversion of angiotensin I to angiotensin II. The resulting reduction in circulating angiotensin II leads to a decrease in BP due to both the loss of the direct vasoconstrictor effect of angiotensin II and decreased aldosterone secretion. ACE inhibitors also act as inhibitors of kininase II, an enzyme that degrades vasodilatory bradykinins. An increase in circulating bradykinins has been postulated as an additional effect of ACE inhibitors that may contribute to the reduction of BP, although current evidence is not conclusive. ACE inhibitors have also been shown to influence other systems involved in the control of BP, including vasopressin release, atrial natriuretic factor release, prostaglandin synthesis, and both sympathetic and parasympathetic nervous system activity [3]. However the relative importance of each of these effects has not been elucidated.

More than 18 different ACE inhibitors have been synthesized [4], with seven currently commercially available (Table 6.1) and more expected to be marketed in the near future. Of these, two have been used extensively in the pediatric age group—captopril and enalapril. Captopril was the first ACE inhibitor to be marketed commercially. Captopril affects the ACE by binding the zinc ion of the enzyme with a sulfhydryl group, thereby deactivating the enzyme. Enalapril uses the same mechanism, but replaces the sulfhydryl group with a carboxyl group. Enalapril is a pro-drug, with the active form, enalaprilat, requiring hepatic transformation after ingestion. Enalaprilat is the only ACE inhibitor approved for intravenous use. Other ACE inhibitors use both modifications of the zinc ligand and the characteristics of biotransformation to alter potency, pharmacokinetics, side effects, and drug interactions. However, no agent has yet proved superior to captopril or enalapril in children.

While numerous studies on the safety and efficacy of ACE inhibitors in adults have been published, such pediatric literature is limited. Captopril is the most widely studied in children and has shown a similar pattern of BP reduction and side effects as that seen in adults [5–9]. Enalapril and its active form enalaprilat are not as well-studied in children, but available literature suggests that they may also be valuable in the treatment of pediatric hypertension [8]. In particular, enalaprilat may be useful in cases where oral medications may not be given, such as in critically ill infants [10].

The side effects of ACE inhibitors in children are similar to those seen in adults (Table 6.2). The most serious of these include renal impairment, hyperkalemia, neutropenia, anemia, and angioedema. The adverse renal effects are most often seen in patients with pre-existing renal insufficiency or renovascular disease. In particular, patients with bilateral renal artery stenosis or with stenosis of the artery to a solitary kidney may develop renal failure. In these conditions of renal artery stenosis, glomerular filtration is maintained, in part, by efferent arteriolar vasoconstriction.

TABLE 6.1
Currently Available Angiotensin-Converting Enzyme Inhibitors

Captopril (Capoten)
Enalapril (Vasotec)
Lisinopril (Prinivil, Zestril)
Fosinopril (Monopril)
Quinapril (Accupril)
Ramipril (Altace)
Benazepril (Lotensin)

TABLE 6.2
Possible Side Effects of Angiotensin-Converting Enzyme Inhibitors

Renal	Proteinuria, renal insufficiency, nephrotic syndrome (contraindicated in bilateral renal artery stenosis), hyperkalemia
Hematologic	Neutropenia, agranulocytosis, anemia, thrombocytopenia, pancytopenia
Cardiovascular	Hypotension, syncope, orthostatic hypotension
Dermatologic	Rash, angioedema, erythema multiforme
Respiratory	Cough, bronchospasm, eosinophilic pneumonitis
Gastrointestinal	Dysgeusia, pancreatitis, glossitis, dyspepsia, jaundice, hepatitis
Central nervous system	Ataxia, confusion, depression
Genitourinary	Impotence

Angiotensin II is responsible for maintaining this vasoconstriction. Reduction of angiotensin II with ACE inhibitors results in relative dilatation of the efferent arterioles, reducing the pressure in the glomerulus necessary for effective glomerular filtration of plasma. While blood flow to the kidney is not reduced, the amount of plasma filtered by the glomerulus is reduced, resulting in azotemia, hyperkalemia, and decreased urine flow. In the absence of pre-existing renal insufficiency or renal artery stenosis, these complications are rare. Indeed, the use of ACE inhibitors in hypertension secondary to unilateral renal artery stenosis is effective in controlling BP. Hematologic complications, while rare, have been seen in children. Routine (1–3 months) monitoring for anemia and neutropenia should be performed. When present, these complications are reversible and improve with discontinuation of the medication. Angioedema is also a rare complication that warrants discontinuing the medication. A dry, nonproductive cough has been reported in 1–5% of patients using ACE inhibitors, although the pediatric literature is limited. It has been postulated that the accumulation of bradykinins caused by the antikininase effect of ACE inhibitors is responsible for cough symptoms. Other reported side effects include hypotension, rash, and diminished taste perception.

The use of ACE inhibitors in pregnancy is contraindicated. Accumulating evidence shows that in the second and third trimesters of pregnancy, maternal use of these drugs has resulted in severe hypotension, anuria, and death in newborns in as many as 20% of cases. It is rare that patients would not respond to other antihypertensive agents during pregnancy; therefore ACE inhibitors should not be used.

The side effects of each particular ACE inhibitor are not well differentiated, with most side effects are relating to the whole class of agents. Newer formulations will attempt to reduce the incidence of side effects, although approval in the pediatric age group will take time. Currently, captopril and enalapril appear to have tolerable side effects when compared with other agents used in the treatment of pediatric hypertension.

The benefits of ACE inhibitors (and calcium channel blockers—see the section below) over other antihypertensive agents are attributed to their negligible adverse effects on lipid profile, carbohydrate metabolism, and cardiac function. These benefits may be particularly important for patients requiring prolonged antihypertensive therapy. Dosages of ACE inhibitors are summarized in Table 6.3.

Calcium Channel Blockers

A mechanism common to all forms of hypertension is increased vascular smooth muscle contractility. As discussed in Chapter 5, calcium influx into smooth muscle cells is essential for contraction. Calcium channel blockers (CCBs) exert their antihypertensive effect by inhibiting the influx of calcium into vascular smooth muscle cells, thus limiting vasoconstriction. In particular, CCBs act primarily as arterial vasodilators by inhibiting calcium influx at voltage-sensitive transmembrane channels. However, these channels are present not only in arterial smooth muscle but in all smooth muscle. The effects of the different types of CCBs, as well as side effects, derive from the relative affinity of these drugs with the calcium channels in various smooth muscle tissues.

There are three major classes of CCBs: phenylalkylamines (verapamil), benzothiazepines (diltiazem), and dihydropyridines (nifedipine, amlodipine, nimodipine, and a variety of newer compounds). Currently available CCBs are listed in Table 6.4. Of these groups, the dihydropyridines are more specific arteriolar vasodilators, while the other two classes have more pronounced effects on cardiac conduction and contractility. Although the nondihydropyridines have a theoretical advantage in treatment of hypertension because their cardiac effects blunt reflex tachycardia, experience in pediatrics is limited primarily to nifedipine for treatment of hypertension. In pediatrics, verapamil has been used to treat supraventric-

TABLE 6.3
Dosages of Angiotensin-Converting Enzyme Inhibitors

	Neonate	*Infant and Child*	*Adolescent and Adult*
Captopril[a]	0.05–0.50 mg/kg/day divided q6–8h	0.5–2.0 mg/kg/day divided q8h	12.5–50.0 mg tid (maximum 200 mg/day)
Enalapril[b]	?	0.1–0.5 mg/kg/day divided q12–24h	2.5–40.0 mg/day divided q12–24h
Enalaprilat[c]	5–10 µg/kg/dose IVq8–24h	Same as for neonates	1.25 mg IV q6h
Lisinopril[d]	?	?	2.5–20.0 mg/day divided q12–24h
Fosinopril[e]	?	?	10–40 mg/day divided q12–24h
Quinapril[f]	?	?	10–80 mg/day divided q12–24h
Ramipril[g]	?	?	2.5–20.0 mg/day divided q12–24h
Benazepril[h]	?	?	10–40 mg/day divided q12–24h

? = dosages for these age groups have not been established.
[a]Available as 12.5-, 25-, 50-, and 100-mg tablets.
[b]Available as 2.5-, 5-, 10-, and 20-mg tablets.
[c]Available as 1.25 mg/ml in 1- and 2-ml vials.
[d]Available as 2.5-, 5-, 10-, 20-, and 40-mg tablets.
[e]Available as 10- and 20-mg tablets.
[f]Available as 5-, 10-, 20-, and 40-mg tablets.
[g]Available as 1.25-, 2.5-, 5-, and 10-mg capsules.
[h]Available as 5-, 10-, 20-, and 40-mg tablets.

TABLE 6.4
Currently Available Calcium Channel Blockers

Phenylalkylamines
    Verapamil (Calan, Calan SR, Isoptin, Isoptin SR, Verelan)
Benzothiazepines
    Diltiazem (Cardizem, Cardizem SR, Cardizem CD, Dilacor XR)
Dihydropyridines
    Nifedipine (Procardia, Procardia XL, Adalat, Adalat CC)
    Nicardipine (Cardene, Cardene SR)
    Isradipine (DynaCirc)
    Nimodipine (Nimotop)
    Felodipine (Plendil Extended-Release)
    Amlodipine (Norvasc)

ular tachycardia [11], and diltiazem has been used in children with pulmonary hypertension [12], muscular dystrophy [13], supraventricular tachycardia [14], and exercise-induced asthma [15]. However, neither drug has been used extensively in pediatric hypertension.

CCBs, like ACE inhibitors, exert little effect on lipid and carbohydrate metabolism and therefore may be superior first-line antihypertensive therapy when compared with other agents such as diuretics or beta-adrenergic antagonists. Unlike ACE inhibitors, CCBs are not contraindicated in patients with renovascular hypertension secondary to bilateral renal artery stenosis or stenosis of the artery to a solitary kidney, nor are they likely to cause further decline of renal function in patients with decreased glomerular filtration rates (GFRs). The effect of CCBs on the kidney is one of afferent arteriolar vasodilation, as opposed to the efferent vasodilation seen with ACE inhibitors [16]. This effect is most pronounced among the dihydropyridines [17]. The selective dilation of afferent arterioles results in increased renal blood flow and enhances glomerular filtration, an effect that may be particularly useful in patients with renovascular hypertension. Whether this effect on the kidney will limit the damage hypertension causes to the kidney remains to be seen, but recent studies suggest that CCBs may exert a protective effect on the kidneys of hypertensive patients [18].

The side effects of CCBs (Table 6.5) are primarily related to inhibition of smooth muscle contraction and vasodilation, and serious side effects are rare. Common side effects include headache, flushing, nausea, constipation, bradycardia (more common with verapamil), ankle edema, and tachycardia.

Most pediatric experiences with CCBs involve the use of nifedipine. Two forms of nifedipine are currently available—a short-acting liquid-filled capsule and a sustained-release formulation. The short-acting preparation is useful in hypertensive emergencies. In adults with pre-existing coronary artery disease, however, long-term use of short-acting nifedipine may be associated with increased mortality [19]. Several studies have shown significant BP reductions in acutely hypertensive children of all ages from newborn to adolescent [11, 20–24]. Side effects of single oral and sublingual doses of 0.25–1.00 mg/kg resulted in few side effects, primarily flushing and tachycardia. No significant episodes of hypotension were reported in any of the studies.

Although the limited dosage forms of the sustained-release formulations (30, 60, and 90 mg) have restricted their use to older children, we have found them to be safe and effective, with the benefit of once or twice daily dosing. The sustained-release formulation acts through a system called the gastrointestinal therapeutic system (GITS) (Procardia XL). The system allows constant release of medication over a prolonged period of time, usually 12–24 hours, providing constant blood levels. The tablet's outer coating is semipermeable, allowing water to enter. A single laser-drilled hole in the outer coating allows release of the drug. Inside the tablet

TABLE 6.5
Side Effects of Calcium Channel Blockers

Common (approximately 10.0%)	Peripheral edema, dizziness, lightheadedness, nausea, headache, flushing, weakness
Less common (approximately 5.0%)	Transient hypotension
Infrequent (<2.0%)	Nasal and chest congestion, dyspnea, diarrhea, constipation, cramps, flatulence, myalgia, muscle cramps, sleep disturbances, blurred vision, rash, urticaria, sexual dysfunction
Rare (<0.5%)	Thrombocytopenia, anemia, leukopenia, allergic hepatitis, gingival hyperplasia, depression, transient blindness

TABLE 6.6
Dosages of Calcium Channel Blockers

	Neonate	*Infant and Child*	*Adolescent and Adult*
Nifedipine[a]	0.25–2.00 mg/kg/dose q6–8h	Same as infant	10–90 mg bid (maximum dose = 180 mg/day)
Verapamil[b]	Contraindicted	4–10 mg/kg/day divided q8h	240–480 mg/day divided q8–12h
Diltiazem[c]	?	?	60–180 bid
Nicardipine[d]	?	?	20–60 mg bid
Isradipine[e]	?	?	2.5–5.0 mg bid
Felodipine[f]	?	?	5–10 mg qd
Amlodipine[g]	?	?	5–10 mg qd

? = dosages for these age groups have not been established.
[a]Available as 10- and 20-mg capsules. For smaller doses, liquid may be aspirated from the capsule with a syringe, with 5.0 mg approximately equal to 0.2 ml of liquid. If the cumulative daily dose exceeds 30 mg, use sustained-release form (Procardia XL: 30-, 60-, and 90-mg sustained-release tablets).
[b]Available as 40-, 80-, and 120-mg capsules, as well as 240-mg sustained-release capsules (Cardizem SR).
[c]Available as Cardizem SR sustained-release capsules (60, 90, and 120 mg).
[d]Available as Cardene SR 30-, 45-, and 60-mg capsules.
[e]Available as DynaCirc 2.5- and 5-mg capsules.
[f]Available as Plendil extended-release 5- and 10-mg capsules.
[g]Available as Norvasc 2.5-, 5-, and 10-mg capsules.

are two layers—a polymer that is hyperosmotic (drawing water into the tablet) and the active drug. As water is osmotically drawn into the tablet, the medication is forced out through the laser-drilled hole, resulting in a controlled release of drug. Recommended pediatric dosages of CCBs are listed in Table 6.6.

TABLE 6.7
Possible Mechanisms of the Antihypertensive Effect of Beta Blockers

---

Decreased cardiac output
Decreased peripheral vascular resistance
Inhibition of renin secretion
Decreased plasma volume
Inhibition of central nervous system sympathetic activity

TABLE 6.8
Distinguishing Characteristics of Various Beta Adrenergic Antagonists

---

Cardioselectivity (beta$_1$-receptor selectivity)
Intrinsic sympathomimetic activity
Alpha-adrenergic antagonism
Membrane-stabilizing effects
Relative hydrophilicity and lipophilicity

Beta-Adrenergic Antagonists

Although numerous beta-adrenergic antagonists (beta blockers) are currently available, the antihypertensive mechanism of this class of drugs is not completely understood. Postulated mechanisms (Table 6.7) vary in their relative importance among the different compounds and are discussed further elsewhere [25].

While all beta blockers inhibit beta-adrenergic receptors throughout the body, they can be distinguished by their activity in several areas (Table 6.8). Cardioselectivity (relative selectivity for beta$_1$-receptors) was developed to minimize the effects of beta blockers on nonvascular beta$_2$-receptors. In particular, bronchoconstriction, impaired glucose tolerance, and alterations in lipid profiles may be reduced with the use of drugs with increased beta$_1$-selectivity.

Intrinsic sympathomimetic activity (ISA) is a partial agonist effect exerted at the beta-receptor by some beta blockers [26]. The theoretical advantages of beta blockers with ISA over drugs without ISA are (1) less depression of left ventricular function, (2) reduced bronchospasm, (3) diminished peripheral vascular compromise, and (4) improved lipid profiles.

Alpha-adrenergic antagonism, in addition to beta-adrenergic antagonism, is a unique property of labetalol. The advantage of alpha-adrenergic antagonism is that it reduces peripheral vascular resistance in addition to the other antihypertensive effects of beta blockers.

The relative hydrophilicity or lipophilicity of each drug affects both gastrointestinal (GI) and CNS absorption. Differences in GI and CNS

TABLE 6.9
Characteristics of Beta-Adrenergic Antagonists

Drug	Cardio-selectivity	ISA	Alpha-Activity	Hydrophilic	Lipophilic
Acebutolol	+	+	−	+	+
Atenolol	+	−	−	+	−
Betaxolol	+	−	−	−	+
Carteolol	−	+	−	+	−
Esmolol	+	−	−	+	−
Labetalol	−	−	+	−	+
Metoprolol	+	−	−	−	+
Nadolol	−	−	−	+	−
Penbutolol	−	+	−	−	+
Pindolol	−	+	−	+	+
Propranolol	−	−	−	−	+
Timolol	−	−	−	+	+

ISA = intrinsic sympathomimetic activity; + = characteristic present in the drug; − = characteristic not present in the drug.

absorption based on relative hydrophilicity/lipophilicity among the different beta blockers may contribute to the incidence of CNS side effects. Manufacturers have attempted to minimize side effects by altering recommended dosage forms and intervals. However, no systematic data exist to clarify which beta blockers are best for a particular patient. When unacceptable CNS side effects occur with a particular beta blocker, it is useful to switch to a beta blocker with a different lipophilicity/hydrophilicity profile. Currently available beta-adrenergic antagonists, as well as information about relative cardioselectivity, ISA, alpha-adrenergic activity, and hydrophilicity and lipophilicity, are listed in Table 6.9.

While the antihypertensive efficacy of beta blockers is well established, they are associated with numerous side effects. Although attempts to modify their chemical properties (see Table 6.9) have improved the tolerability of beta blockers, fewer side effects are seen with both ACE inhibitors and CCBs, thereby favoring their use as first-line medications. Side effects of beta blockers are summarized in Table 6.10.

Beta blockers are contraindicated in patients with asthma, insulin-dependent diabetes mellitus, Raynaud's phenomenon, congestive heart failure, and atrioventricular conduction disturbances other than first-degree heart block. Patients with pre-existing cardiovascular disease may experience severe reactions to abrupt withdrawal, including exacerbation of pre-existing angina, myocardial infarction, or sudden death. In children, blunting of the normal response to hypoglycemia (e.g., release of catecholamines, stimulation of glycogenolysis, gluconeogenesis, and lipolysis) may be particularly significant [27]. Children with decreased oral intake,

TABLE 6.10
Side Effects of Beta Blockers

Cardiovascular effects	Bradycardia, hypotension, syncope, shock, exacerbation of angina pectoris in susceptible patients, fluid retention
Central nervous system effects	Lightheadedness, ataxia, dizziness, irritability, sleepiness, hearing loss, visual disturbances, vivid dreams/nightmares, hallucinations, weakness, fatigue, depression
Gastrointestinal effects	Nausea, vomiting, diarrhea, cramping, constipation, flatulence
Hematologic effects	Transient eosinophilia, idiosyncratic reactions of thrombocytopenia, nonthrombocytopenic purpura, agranulocytosis
Other effects	Impotence, rash

TABLE 6.11
Recommended Dosages of Several Beta Blockers

	Children	*Adults*
Propranolol*	0.5–2.0 mg/kg/day q6–12h (maximum 8 mg/kg/day)	Initial: 40 mg/dose bid (maximum 480 mg/day)
Nadolol	?	40–160 mg/day (once daily)
Atenolol	?	50–100 mg/day (once daily)
Metoprolol	?	100–200 mg/day (once or twice daily)
Acebutolol	?	200–800 mg/day (once daily)
Labetalol	?	100–400 mg/day bid

*Available as tablets—10, 20, 40, 60, 80, and 90 mg; as extended-release capsules—60, 80, 120, and 160 mg; and as suspensions—20, 40, and 80 mg/ml.

either secondary to illness or for medical reasons (e.g., NPO for surgery), who are using beta blockers should be followed closely.

Pediatric experience with beta blockers has accumulated since the first reports of the use of propranolol in children and adolescents in the 1970s [28, 29]. A variety of childhood diseases other than hypertension (i.e., arrhythmias, hypertrophic cardiomyopathy, tetralogy of Fallot, mitral valve prolapse, Marfan's syndrome, Bartter's syndrome, thyrotoxicosis, and migraine prophylaxis) have also been treated with beta blockers [27]. The wide use of these agents in children has allowed determinations of safe and effective dosing. However, many of the newer agents with diminished side effects and more specific actions are not available in convenient pediatric formulations. Pediatric dosages for propranolol, atenolol, labetalol, and metoprolol have been recommended [30, 31]. Table 6.11 lists several beta blockers and recommended dosages.

Diuretics

Diuretics have long been considered safe, effective, and inexpensive first-line therapy for hypertension. With the development of beta blockers, ACE inhibitors, and CCBs, the primacy of diuretics has been challenged. The accumulated experience with diuretics far exceeds that of the newer classes of drugs, and the value of each new medication can be compared with these well-studied agents.

Diuretics, particularly thiazides, were once the drug of first choice in the therapy of mild to moderate hypertension. While the trend is toward increasing use of ACE inhibitors, CCBs, and beta blockers as first-line therapy, several authors have questioned the replacement of diuretics [32]. Arguments against the use of diuretics have focused on their alterations in lipid and glucose metabolism, as well as the question of whether their use prevents the long-term sequelae of hypertension (e.g., stroke, myocardial infarction, sudden cardiac death, and atherosclerotic heart disease). Although initial reports of the newer agents appear to favor their use, more definitive initial therapy of hypertension awaits clinical experience similar to that of diuretics.

Although diuretics have been used to treat a variety of conditions from congestive heart failure to hypercalciuria, our discussion is limited to treatment of hypertension. Despite more than 30 years of experience, the precise mechanisms by which diuretics reduce BP are unclear. Reduction of extracellular fluid volume and sodium chloride play a role. Like patients who respond to dietary salt restriction, there is a subset of hypertensive patients who have an enhanced response to diuretic therapy when compared with other patients. Blacks, the elderly, and patients with low-renin forms of hypertension are included in this subset. The relationship between sodium and intravascular volume depletion as a mechanism for the antihypertensive effect of diuretics is indicated by the fact that dietary salt supplementation can reverse the effects of diuretics [33, 34]. Further evidence that the antihypertensive effects of salt restriction and diuretic therapy share a common mechanism is reviewed in detail elsewhere [35]. Others have suggested that diuretics may also exert a direct vasodilatory effect [36, 37], although the evidence is not as clear.

All diuretics exert action on the kidney by inhibiting the absorption of solute, resulting in decreased reabsorption of water and subsequent increased urine flow. Diuretics are classified by the mechanisms with which inhibition of solute reabsorption is accomplished. Figure 6.1 shows the various parts of the nephron and the sites of action of the various diuretics. Combinations of diuretics with different sites of action can increase efficacy. For example, in patients with decreased GFRs, the addition of metolazone to furosemide increases sodium delivery to the loop of Henle, thus effectively increasing diuresis. Osmotic diuretics (mannitol) and carbonic anhydrase inhibitors are not effective in the therapy of hypertension and are not discussed further here.

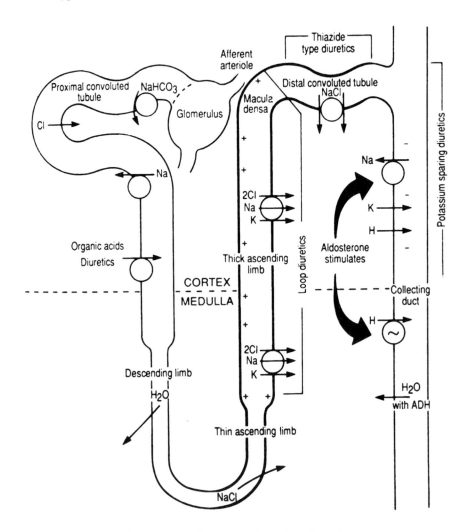

FIGURE 6.1. Sites of action of diuretics. (Reproduced with permission from MS Pecker. Pathophysiologic Effects and Strategies for Long-Term Diuretic Treatment of Hypertension. In JH Laragh, BM Brenner [eds], Hypertension: Pathophysiology, Diagnosis, and Management. New York: Raven, 1990;2145.)

The role of diuretics as adjunctive therapy with other drugs is clear. Improved BP control is noted in patients treated with diuretics combined with ACE inhibitors, CCBs, and beta blockers. Table 6.12 lists dosages of commonly used diuretics.

Table 6.13 summarizes the major side effects of the various diuretic agents. More detailed reviews of the pharmacokinetics of diuretics in neonates [38, 39] and older children [40] have been published.

TABLE 6.12
Recommended Dosages of Commonly Used Diuretics

	Child	*Adult*
Chlorothiazide[a]	5–10 mg/kg/dose bid	0.25–1.00 g/dose qd–bid
Hydrochlorothiazide[b]	0.5–2.0 mg/kg/dose qd–bid	25–100 mg/dose qd–bid
Furosemide[c]	0.5–2.0 mg/kg/dose qd–qid	Same as children
Bumetanide[d]	?	0.5–2.0 mg/dose
Spironolactone[e]	1–3 mg/kg/day bid–qid	25–100 mg/day bid–qid
Metolazone[f]	0.2–0.4 mg/kg/day qd–bid	2.5–5.0 mg/dose qd–bid

[a]Available as 250- and 500-mg tablets, and as 250 mg/5 ml oral suspension.
[b]Available as 25-, 50-, and 100-mg tabs, and as 50 mg/5 ml and 100 mg/ml oral solutions.
[c]Available as 20-, 40-, and 80-mg tablets, and as 10 mg/ml oral solutions.
[d]Available as 0.5-, 1-, and 2-mg tablets.
[e]Available as 25-, 50-, and 100-mg tabs, and as 2 mg/ml oral suspension.
[f]Available as 2.5-, 5.0-, and 10.0-mg tabs, and as 0.1 mg/ml oral suspension.

TABLE 6.13
Summary of Major Side Effects of Diuretic Agents

	Loop	*Thiazide*	*Potassium-Sparing*
Hypokalemia	Yes	Yes	No
Hyperkalemia	No	No	Yes
Hypercalciuria	Yes	No	No
Hyperuricemia	Yes	Yes	No
Hypomagnesemia	Yes	Yes	No
Hyperglycemia	No	Yes	Possible
Hyperlipidemia	No	Yes	No

Thiazide Diuretics

The thiazide (benzothiadiazide) diuretics (hydrochlorothiazide, chlorothiazide, chlorthalidone, metolazone) have been used extensively for pediatric hypertension [38–40], with most experience involving hydrochlorothiazide and chlorothiazide. They are members of the sulfonamide class of drugs and are poorly filtered at the glomerulus. They enter the nephron primarily by transport into the proximal convoluted tubule via organic acid transport mechanisms. Once in the tubule, they are believed to inhibit sodium chloride transporters in the luminal membrane of the distal convoluted tubule, resulting in increased sodium delivery to the distal nephron and increased loss of free water. In addition to blocking reabsorption of sodium and chloride, they also influence excretion of calcium (increasing reabsorption), magnesium, and potassium (increasing uri-

TABLE 6.14
Side Effects of Thiazide Diuretics

Fluid and electrolyte disturbances	Hypokalemia, volume depletion and hypotension, hypomagnesemia, hypercalcemia
Metabolic disturbances	Decreased glucose tolerance, hyperlipidemia, hyperuricemia
Gastrointestinal	Anorexia, gastric irritation, nausea and vomiting, cramping, diarrhea, intrahepatic cholestatic jaundice, pancreatitis
Neurologic	Dizziness, vertigo, headache, paresthesia
Hematologic (rare)	Leukopenia, thrombocytopenic purpura, agranulocytosis, aplastic anemia
Other	Photosensitivity, rash, urticaria, toxic epidermal necrolysis

nary losses). Their antihypertensive effect, as discussed above, is probably related to depletion of intravascular volume and is enhanced by dietary salt restriction.

The decreased use of thiazides as first-line antihypertensive treatment relates to their side effects (Table 6.14). In children, thiazides have been shown to displace bilirubin from binding sites of albumin [41] and should therefore be used with caution in neonates with hyperbilirubinemia. Hypokalemia is the most potentially dangerous side effect of thiazides; therefore serum potassium should be monitored at regular intervals after initiation of therapy. The significance of alterations in glucose metabolism and lipid profiles has not been systematically examined in children, and it is not clear whether these disturbances are sufficient to preclude use of thiazides as first-line antihypertensive drugs.

Loop Diuretics

The loop diuretics (furosemide, bumetanide, ethacrynic acid) inhibit reabsorption of sodium (and chloride) in the thick ascending limb of Henle's loop. A likely mechanism involves inhibition of a luminal Na-K-2Cl cotransporter that increases distal tubular delivery of sodium chloride. As with the thiazides, this results in a free-water diuresis. The loop diuretics are the most potent diuretics and are useful in the short-term treatment of hypertension related to acute fluid overload (such as acute glomerulonephritis). Also, in patients with decreased renal function (GFR <10 ml/min/1.73 m^2), they are more effective than thiazide diuretics. The side effects of loop diuretics are almost identical to those of the thiazides (see Table 6.14). However, unlike thiazides, which increase calcium reabsorption from the distal nephron, loop diuretics produce hypercalciuria. Thus chronic use can lead to nephrocalcinosis and nephrolithiasis. Like thiazides, loop diuretics displace bilirubin from albumin and therefore should be used with caution in neonates. Also, ototoxicity has been reported in patients receiving furosemide, particularly when combined with other oto-toxic medications [42, 43].

Potassium-Sparing Diuretics

The third group of diuretics that have been used in the treatment of hyper-tension (although on a more limited scale) are the potassium-sparing diuretics (spironolactone, triamterene, amiloride). They are the least potent of the three groups and are used primarily when use of other diuret-ics is needed, but would result in hypokalemia.

Spironolactone exerts its diuretic effect by acting as a competitive antagonist of aldosterone. The diuretic effect is based on decreased reab-sorption of sodium, chloride, and water in the collecting duct, resulting in increased reabsorption of potassium, ammonium, phosphate, and titratable acid. It is most effective in states of elevated plasma aldosterone (e.g., hyperaldosteronism, congestive heart failure, and hepatic disease). It is rel-atively ineffective in conditions of normal plasma aldosterone. When used alone, spironolactone has a mild antihypertensive effect. This effect is enhanced when combined with thiazide or loop diuretics. Amiloride and triamterene have not been used extensively in the treatment of pediatric hypertension. Amiloride may be of particular value in patients with rare forms of glucocorticoid-remediable hypertension.

Direct Vasodilators

Although they are discussed together here, the direct vasodilators are structurally unrelated, acting through a variety of mechanisms to directly relax vascular smooth muscle and decrease BP [44]. This section discusses hydralazine, minoxidil, diazoxide, and nitroprusside. These drugs are pri-marily used to treat hypertensive urgencies and emergencies. Long-term effectiveness of these drugs has been limited by the body's compensatory responses to their actions (e.g., increased cardiac output and fluid reten-tion), by development of tolerance, and by side effects (Table 6.15). Thus, despite their value in the emergency situations, their use as chronic anti-hypertensive medications is limited to only the most refractory cases. In such cases, concurrent therapy with a beta blocker, a diuretic, or both is often necessary.

Hydralazine

Hydralazine primarily acts to vasodilate the arteriolar resistance vessels. Its effect on the venous capacitance vessels is less pronounced. The mechanism is unclear. Postulated mechanisms include modulation of cyclic adenosine monophosphate–mediated vasodilation [45], interaction with endothelial-related vasodilatory factors [46], or some other unidenti-

TABLE 6.15
Common Side Effects of Direct Vasodilators

Headache
Palpitations
Tachycardia
Flushing
Fluid and sodium retention
Precipitation of angina in susceptible patients

fied mechanism. In the acute cases of hypertension, hydralazine is an effective antihypertensive. It is available in both oral and intravenous forms. Its onset of action is approximately 30–60 minutes after dosing. The delay in the onset of action when compared with other vasodilators should be noted, and additional doses should be delayed until the initial dose has been allowed to exert its action. Chronic use of hydralazine is usually limited to those cases in which single- and two-drug regimens have failed. When used, it is often necessary to combine it with a diuretic and a beta blocker.

In addition to the side effects common to other direct vasodilators, hydralazine has unique adverse effects. In as many as 10% of patients, a syndrome resembling systemic lupus erythematosus or rheumatoid arthritis has been reported. Patients may have fever, arthralgia, splenomegaly, lymphadenopathy, myalgia, pleuritic chest pain, and edema. Laboratory evaluation reveals antinuclear antibodies and possibly anti–single-stranded DNA antibodies (as opposed to the anti–double-stranded DNA antibodies seen in traditional SLE). The syndrome is resolved after discontinuation of hydralazine, but it may take several weeks. Hydralazine is contraindicated in patients with coronary artery disease, cerebrovascular disorders, and mitral valve heart disease, as well as in patients who have demonstrated hypersensitivity to the drug.

Hydralazine has been used safely in children [47–49]. No side effects different from those in the adult literature have been reported. The lupus-like syndrome has been reported in a 9-year–old girl [50] and an infant [51] whose mother had received hydralazine while pregnant. Dosages are listed in Table 6.16. Hydralazine is available in liquid, tablet, and intravenous forms, which facilitates dosing in younger children.

Minoxidil

Minoxidil, like hydralazine, vasodilates primarily the arteriolar resistance vessels. The exact mechanism of the vasodilatory effect of minoxidil is unknown. Suggested mechanisms of action include the following: (1) K^+-channel agonist activity, causing opening of potassium channels in vascu-

TABLE 6.16
Recommended Dosages of Direct Vasodilators

	Children	*Adults*
Hydralazine[a]	PO: 0.5–2.0 mg/kg/dose bid–qid	10–50 mg/dose qid
	IV: 0.1–0.5 mg/kg/dose q4–6h	Same
Minoxidil[b]	PO: 0.1–0.5 mg/kg/dose qd–bid	2.5–20.0 mg/dose qd–bid
Diazoxide	IV: 1–2 mg/kg/dose q10mins until response (max dose in 24 hours = 10 mg/kg	Same
Nitroprusside	IV: 0.5–8.0 μg/kg/min continuous infusion	Same

[a]Available as 10-, 25-, 50-, and 100-mg tablets; 0.2 mg/ml oral liquid; and 20 mg/ml injection.
[b]Available as 2.5- and 10.0-mg tablets.

TABLE 6.17
Possible Side Effects of Minoxidil*

Salt and fluid retention
Congestive heart failure
Pericardial effusion/pericardial tamponade
Tachycardia
Exacerbation of angina pectoris
Hirsutism

*In addition to the side effects listed in Table 6.15.

lar smooth muscle, leading to hyperpolarization and decreased contractility [52]; and (2) modulation of cyclic adenosine monophosphate– or cyclic guanosine monophosphate (GMP)–mediated vasodilation [44].

Minoxidil is a very effective vasodilator. However, because of an unfavorable side effect profile, it is not used in first- or second-line therapy of hypertension. Current use is limited to patients who are refractory to treatment with maximal doses of two other classes of antihypertensive medications and a diuretic, or to patients who cannot tolerate other classes of medications. It is effective in patients with renal impairment. Use of minoxidil almost uniformly requires concurrent use of a diuretic and a beta blocker because of fluid and sodium retention and reflex adrenergic stimulation.

In addition to the side effects common to all vasodilators, several unique properties of minoxidil should be noted (Table 6.17). Sodium and fluid retention are a particularly marked effect of minoxidil. Pericardial effusion and congestive heart failure have resulted. Hypertrichosis is common and is often a reason for poor compliance. Hypertrichosis is a reversible effect and resolves after discontinuation of the drug. Contraindications to the use of minoxidil include presence or suspicion of pheochromocytoma, congestive heart failure, recent myocardial infarction, and hypersensitivity to the drug.

Minoxidil has been used effectively in children [53–55]. Effective BP reduction can be obtained in children whose hypertension is refractory to multiple-drug regimens. Side effects parallel those seen in adults, with fluid retention and pericardial effusion reported in most patients, and hypertrichosis occuring almost universally in pediatric patients. In cases of severe, refractory hypertension, minoxidil remains an effective oral medication. We recommend that treatment be initiated in the inpatient setting, with close observation for signs of fluid overload. Dosage recommendations are listed in Table 6.16.

Diazoxide

Diazoxide is a benzothiadiazide but shares none of the diuretic effects of the other thiazides discussed above. In fact, use of diazoxide, like use of other direct vasodilators, results in a significant antidiuresis. It is an extremely powerful vasodilator that, like hydralazine and minoxidil, selectively dilates the arteriolar resistance vessels more than the venous capacitance vessels. The mechanism of this action is unknown.

The use of intravenous diazoxide is limited to hypertensive emergencies. Its onset of action is rapid, and sometimes unpredictable, resulting in significant hypotension. For this reason, other agents should be used as primary therapy for hypertensive emergencies (see the section on hypertensive emergencies). Diazoxide should be reserved for patients who do not respond to other therapy, or for those patients in whom immediate BP reduction is needed (e.g., because of hypertensive encephalopathy). Because of significant fluid retention, concurrent use of diuretics is recommended. While oral forms of diazoxide exist, they are primarily used for treatment of chronic hypoglycemic states, and there is no role for oral diazoxide in the treatment of pediatric hypertension.

In addition to the previously discussed adverse effects of direct vasodilators (e.g., fluid and sodium retention, reflex tachycardia, and sympathetic discharge), there are several important adverse effects unique to diazoxide (Table 6.18). Hyperglycemia is common (>5%) when diazoxide is used for longer than 3 days and may occur sooner. It is contraindicated when a rapid reduction in BP may be detrimental, as with intracerebral hemorrhage, dissecting aortic aneurysm, acute myocardial infarction, and aortic coarctation.

Although diazoxide was previously felt to be the agent of choice in pediatric hypertensive emergencies, more recent experience with CCBs [11], beta blockers [56], and sodium nitroprusside (see the following section) favors their use.

TABLE 6.18
Possible Side Effects of Diazoxide*

Metabolic	Hyperglycemia, hyperuricemia
Cardiovascular	Hypotension, fluid overload, edema, congestive heart failure, angina, arrhythmias
Gastrointestinal	Nausea, vomiting, constipation
Miscellaneous	Hypertrichosis, local effects at injection site (burning, cellulitis), skin rash, fever, leukopenia, thrombocytopenia

*In addition to the side effects listed in Table 6.15.

Nitroprusside

Nitroprusside (sodium nitroprusside) differs from the other vasodilators because of its primary effect on venous capacitance vessels at low doses. At commonly used therapeutic doses, nitroprusside equally affects both venous capacitance and arteriolar resistance vessels [57]. The mechanism of action is related to formation of an endothelial-derived relaxation factor (EDRF), identified as nitric oxide [58, 59]. Nitric oxide causes relaxation of vascular smooth muscles by binding to guanylyl cyclase, an enzyme that increases both intracellular concentrations of cyclic GMP and subsequent relaxation of the smooth muscle cells. It is unclear whether nitroprusside serves as a substrate for formation of nitric oxide or is converted to some other substance that also serves to activate guanylyl cyclase [60].

Nitroprusside is an immediate-acting intravenous antihypertensive to be used in hypertensive emergencies. Because of its rapid metabolism, it must be given as a continuous infusion. The response is largely dosage-dependent, and continuous infusion permits accurate titration of effect. Use of nitroprusside requires frequent monitoring of BP, with arterial monitoring preferred. Once BP has been controlled with nitroprusside, either the cause of hypertension should be treated or other antihypertensives should be started, in an attempt to minimize the duration of nitroprusside treatment.

An important side effect of nitroprusside treatment is accumulation of the toxic metabolites cyanide and thiocyanate. In patients requiring prolonged therapy (>24 hours), thiocyanate levels should be monitored daily. Accumulation of toxic metabolites is more common in patients with renal and hepatic insufficiency. Signs of cyanide toxicity include anxiety, headache, dizziness, confusion, jaw stiffness, seizures, and a bitter almond odor to the breath. Additionally, laboratory studies may show metabolic acidosis and hypoxemia. Other side effects of nitroprusside therapy are listed in Table 6.19.

Nitroprusside is contraindicated when hypertension is related to a compensatory state (e.g., coarctation of the aorta) or in patients with

TABLE 6.19
Possible Side Effects of Nitroprusside Use

Hypotension (particular attention should be paid to infusion rate and delivery
   system for errors)
Cyanide toxicity
Methemoglobinemia
Systemic symptoms (i.e., anorexia, nausea, abdominal cramps, diaphoresis,
   headache, chills)
Hypothyroidism
Tinnitus
Visual disturbances

---

increased intracranial pressure. Nitroprusside has been effective in pediatric hypertensive emergencies, using the same precautions for hypotension and cyanide toxicity as those used for adults. Infusion should begin at 0.3 µg/kg/minute and be increased as necessary to a maximum of 8.0 µg/kg/minute. Average dosages are approximately 3.0 µg/kg/minute. At dosages of greater than 8.0 µg/kg/minute, the risk of cyanide toxicity surpasses the possible benefits of therapy, and nitroprusside should be discontinued. In patients with renal insufficiency, concurrent peritoneal or hemodialysis may be used to limit cyanide toxicity. Recommended dosages of direct vasodilators are summarized in Table 6.16.

Central Nervous System Sympathetic Inhibitors

Evidence that increased CNS sympathetic activity is a characteristic of some forms of hypertension [61] has supported development of a class of drugs known alternatively as centrally acting sympathetic inhibitors, centrally acting alpha-agonists, centrally acting sympatholytic agents, or central sympatholytics. Clonidine, methyldopa, guanabenz, and guanfacine are examples of CNS sympathetic inhibitors.

Observations of increased CNS sympathetic activity related to BP include the following:

1.   Resting heart rate, cardiac output, and oxygen consumption are elevated in some hypertensives [61].
2.   Stress can increase BP. Meditation and biofeedback can reduce BP [62].
3.   In some patients with labile hypertension there is a positive correlation between diastolic BP and plasma norepinephrine levels [63].
4.   Elevated cerebrospinal fluid norepinephrine levels have been seen in essential hypertension [63].
5.   Left ventricular hypertrophy in hypertension may be mediated in part by circulating catecholamine levels [64].

TABLE 6.20
Benefits of Central Sympatholytic Drugs

Decrease in left ventricular mass
Stable or improved lipid profiles
Preserved renal hemodynamics
No clinically important alteration in glucose metabolism

TABLE 6.21
Side Effects of Central Sympatholytic Drugs

Sedation
Dry mouth
Depression, vivid dreams/nightmares, hallucinations
Impotence, decreased libido, ejaculatory difficulty
Rebound hypertension when discontinued abruptly

Consistent with the evidence of increased CNS sympathetic activity in hypertension, drugs that inhibit central sympathetic activity are effective antihypertensives. The mechanism of action of the central sympatholytic agents is based on modulation of CNS centers for cardiovascular control. In the dorsal medulla, the nucleus of the tractus solitarius coordinates afferent signals from various baroreceptors and sends out efferent signals to the ventrolateral medulla. Stimulation of $alpha_2$-adrenergic receptors in the ventrolateral medulla by endogenous catecholamines (or their agonists) results in decreased peripheral sympathetic activity. The resulting decrease in cardiac output, heart rate, and total peripheral resistance (and possibly a drug-induced inhibition of renin release) leads to a reduction in BP. More complex mechanisms are also involved and have been reviewed [61, 63, 65], but inhibition of CNS sympathetic output by stimulation of CNS $alpha_2$-adrenergic receptors can account for the antihypertensive effects of clonidine, methyldopa, guanfacine, and guanabenz.

Despite their efficacy as antihypertensive medications, central sympatholytics are frequently being replaced by newer classes of drugs with fewer side effects. However, because of their unique mechanism of action, they may have benefits not seen in other classes of drugs (Table 6.20). The reduction in left ventricular mass and favorable lipid profiles, in addition to their acceptable use in patients with renal failure and diabetes mellitus, suggest that more widespread use of these agents would be beneficial.

However, significant side effects are seen at dosages needed to treat hypertension (Table 6.21). The high incidence of side effects results in poor compliance. When patients discontinue treatment, a discontinuation syndrome often results, with BPs returning to values at or above pretreatment levels, occasionally precipitating a hypertensive crisis. Newer forms of the drugs, including transdermal clonidine and long-acting guanfacine, may improve the side effect profile. Such forms are discussed below.

Pediatric experience with CNS sympathetic inhibitors is limited. Some reports discussing behavior problems [66, 67] have been published, although no clear relationship has been found. Side effects and toxicity are similar to those reported in adults [68–70]. Despite their antihypertensive efficacy, the frequency of side effects and the dangers of accidental ingestions preclude the use of central sympatholytics as first-line therapy in children. Exceptions include children in whom CCBs, ACE inhibitors, and beta blockers are contraindicated or ineffective, and patients for whom compliance is a major problem and who may benefit from the simplicity of the transdermal clonidine patch.

Clonidine

Clonidine acts as an agonist of CNS alpha-adrenoceptors (primarily alpha$_2$). When initial doses are given, a transient increase in BP is often seen, suggesting that clonidine also stimulates peripheral (vasoconstrictive) alpha-receptors, although central sympatholytic activity ultimately predominates. In addition to the side effects experienced with all CNS sympathetic inhibitors, effects unique to clonidine are rare and include transient elevations of liver enzymes, muscle or joint pain, weight gain, and rash. Oral dosages are listed in Table 6.22.

A transdermal clonidine preparation is also available. This formulation allows sustained release of clonidine through a patch. Patches are available that give 0.1, 0.2, or 0.3 mg/day dosage equivalents. Steady-state levels are reached after 48–72 hours, and patches are changed weekly. Theoretical benefits of this preparation include stable blood levels of medication over time, resulting in fewer side effects and reduction in the incidence of discontinuation hypertension. Irritant or allergic skin reactions are seen in 15–20% of patients and occasionally require discontinuation of therapy. Cross-sensitivity to oral clonidine after allergic reactions to the patch has been reported.

Methyldopa

Methyldopa is metabolized to methylnorepinephrine. In addition to stimulation of CNS alpha$_2$-adrenergic receptors, other antihypertensive actions have been proposed. For example, methyldopa (as methylnorepinephrine) may displace norepinephrine from stores in adrenergic nerve endings and act as a false neurotransmitter at peripheral alpha-receptors, blunting the vasoconstrictive effect of peripheral alpha-adrenoceptor stimulation. However, CNS effects are thought to be the most important [65].

Methyldopa is associated with both a higher incidence of fluid retention and weight gain and a less favorable effect on lipid profile than the other central sympatholytics. In approximately 25% of patients taking methyl-

TABLE 6.22
Recommended Dosages of Central Sympatholytic Agents

Agents	Children	Adults
Clonidine[a]	0.05–0.30 mg/dose bid–tid	0.1–0.6 mg/dose bid
Methyldopa[b]	5–20 mg/kg/dose bid–tid	250–1,000 mg/dose bid
Guanabenz[c]	?	4–16 mg/dose bid
Guanfacine[d]	?	1–3 mg/dose qd

[a]Available as 0.1- and 0.2-mg tablets and as patch transdermal therapeutic system (TTS) 1 (0.1 mg), TTS 2 (0.2 mg), and TTS 3 (0.3 mg).
[b]Available as 125-, 250-, and 500-mg tablets, and 250 mg/5 ml oral suspension.
[c]Available as 4- and 8-mg tablets.
[d]Available as 1- and 2-mg tablets.

dopa, a positive direct Coomb's reaction develops, with auto-antibody developed against the Rh antigens. Of these patients, about 5% develop hemolytic anemia or hepatitis, requiring discontinuation of the drug. Positive antinuclear antibody, rheumatoid factor, and lupus erythematosus serology have also been reported, but clinical manifestations are rare. Dosages are listed in Table 6.22.

Guanabenz

The antihypertensive mechanism of guanabenz is similar to that of clonidine—stimulation of CNS alpha-adrenoceptors resulting in decreased central sympathetic discharge to peripheral sites. It is more selective for alpha$_2$-adrenoceptors, although the clinical significance of this property is unknown. Guanabenz reduces serum cholesterol and low-density lipoprotein concentrations [71] and causes the least amount of fluid retention of the class. Side effects are similar to side effects of other sympatholytics. Dosages are listed in Table 6.22.

Guanfacine

Guanfacine is the newest of the centrally acting sympatholytics. Its mechanism of action is similar to that of clonidine and guanabenz, but it has a longer half-life permitting once-daily dosing. Side effects are also similar to clonidine and guanabenz, although reportedly less frequent.

Miscellaneous Antihypertensive Medications

Reserpine

Reserpine is derived from the plant *Rauwolfia serpentina* and is a member of a class of drugs known as rauwolfia alkaloids. It acts to reduce BP

TABLE 6.23
Possible Side Effects of Reserpine

Central nervous system	Depression (contraindicated in patients with clinical depression), sedation, lethargy, weakness, decreased libido, impotence, nightmares, anxiety, headache
Gastrointestinal	Increased motility and secretion, increased risk of gastric ulceration, increased appetite, weight gain, nausea, vomiting, diarrhea
Cardiovascular	Hypotension, fluid retention, syncope, chest pain, arrhythmias
Respiratory	Bronchospasm, dyspnea
Hematologic	Purpura, epistaxis, thrombocytopenia
Other	Menorrhagia, nasal congestion, gynecomastia, arthralgia, myalgia, rash, pruritus

through a reduction in sympathetic nervous system activity; however its mechanism of action is different from the alpha- and beta-receptor agonists and antagonists discussed above. Reserpine blocks the physiologic reuptake of dopamine into the chromaffin granules of nerve endings. The conversion of dopamine into norepinephrine in the chromaffin granules is thus blocked. Stores of neurotransmitters, particularly catecholamines and 5-hydroxytryptamine, in the nerve endings of sympathetic nerves are depleted. Catecholamine depletion occurs in many tissues throughout the body, including brain, adrenal medulla, myocardium, blood vessels, and adrenergic nerve terminals.

Reserpine is an effective antihypertensive medication, particularly when used with a diuretic. However, the presence of significant side effects (Table 6.23) and the existence of more effective drugs precludes its use in most cases of pediatric hypertension. Increased appetite, weight gain, depression, and nasal congestion are seen in more than 5% of cases, resulting in poor compliance. Pediatric dosage is 0.01–0.02 mg/kg/day. It is available in a 0.05 mg/ml elixir and as 0.10- and 0.25-mg tablets.

Prazosin

Prazosin is representative of a class of antihypertensive drugs that act through selective antagonism of peripheral alpha$_1$-adrenergic receptors (others include terazosin, doxazosin, trimazosin, indoramin). Through blockade of vascular alpha$_1$-receptors, these drugs dilate both arteriolar resistance and venous capacitance vessels. Unlike the direct vasodilators discussed above, prazosin and related compounds cause less reflex tachycardia, renin release, and catecholamine excretion. A disadvantage is the common occurrence of postural hypotension, particularly with the initial dosage. The first dosage should be given in the evening, and patients

TABLE 6.24
Possible Side Effects of Prazosin

Common (>5%)	Dizziness, headache, drowsiness, decreased energy, weakness, palpitations, nausea
Less frequent (1–4%)	Vomiting, diarrhea, constipation, edema, orthostatic hypotension, dyspnea, syncope, vertigo, depression, rash, urinary frequency, blurred vision, reddened sclerae, epistaxis, nasal congestion
Rare (<1%)	Abdominal pain, pancreatitis, liver function abnormalities, tachycardia, paresthesia, hallucinations, pruritus, alopecia, urinary incontinence, impotence, priapism, tinnitus

should be warned that significant hypotension, tachycardia, and syncope may occur but usually improve after subsequent dosages. Additional side effects are listed in Table 6.24.

Prazosin is an effective antihypertensive, although pediatric experience is limited. In our experience, prazosin is of limited value. There have been no reports of glucose abnormalities, and a favorable effect on lipid profiles has been reported with doxazosin [72]. Prazosin may be useful as a second- or third-line drug in patients with either diabetes or renal insufficiency. An extended release form is available (prazosin GITS), although there is no published pediatric experience. The initial adult dose is 1 mg tid. It is available in 1-, 2-, and 5-mg tablets. No specific pediatric dosages have been established.

Phenoxybenzamine and Phentolamine

Both phenoxybenzamine and phentolamine are alpha-adrenergic antagonists. Because of their side effects and the availability of other drugs, their use is limited to treatment of pheochromocytoma. Phentolamine is used intravenously, primarily during acute hypertensive crises of pheochromocytoma or before surgery in which catecholamine excess is expected. Phenoxybenzamine is an orally available medication used for chronic therapy of pheochromocytoma. Because reflex tachycardia is common, concurrent use with a beta-adrenergic antagonist is often necessary. Both drugs are discussed below in the section on treatment of pheochromocytoma.

Future Medications

Current antihypertensive drugs act on a variety of the body's mechanisms of BP control. Ongoing research will clarify the role of each of these medica-

TABLE 6.25
Contraindications to the Use of Various Antihypertensive Medications

---

Angiotensin-converting enzyme inhibitors
  Pregnancy
  Bilateral renal artery stenosis (or renal artery stenosis in solitary kidney)
  Acute renal failure
Calcium channel blockers
  Left ventricular dysfunction (verapamil and diltiazem)
  Sick sinus syndrome, second- or third-degree atrioventricular block (verapamil
    and diltiazem)
  Atrial flutter or atrial fibrillation (verapamil and diltiazem)
  Neonates (verapamil and diltiazem)
Beta-adrenergic antagonists
  Asthma
  Insulin-dependent diabetes mellitus
  Raynaud's phenomenon
  Congestive heart failure
  Atrioventricular conduction disturbances (other than first degree heart block)
Diuretics
  Thiazides—hyperbilirubinemia in neonates
  Loop—hypercalciuria/nephrocalcinosis
  Potassium sparing—hyperkalemia, diabetic nephropathy
Direct vasodilators
  Hydralazine—coronary artery disease, cerebrovascular disease, mitral valve disease
  Minoxidil—pheochromocytoma, congestive heart failure, recent myocardial
    infarction
  Diazoxide—cerebral hemorrhage, dissecting aortic aneurysm, acute myocardial
    infarction, aortic coarctation
  Nitroprusside—coarctation of aorta, increased intracranial pressure
Central sympathetic inhibitors
  Clonidine, guanabenz, guanfacine—only hypersensitivity to drug
  Methyldopa—acute/active hepatic disease
Other drugs
  Reserpine—mental depression
  Prazosin—only hypersensitivity to drug

---

tions, as well as formulate new compounds that maximize antihypertensive efficacy while minimizing side effects. Newer agents that act on other aspects of BP control are under development and include both potassium channel openers (pinacidil, cromakalim, lemakalim) and renin antagonists.

Table 6.25 summarizes contraindictions to the use of various antihypertensive medications. Table 6.26 summarizes important pharmacokinetic properties of the most commonly used antihypertensive medications. This table may be used to maximize antihypertensive efficacy in patients requiring multiple medications.

TABLE 6.26
Pharmacodynamics of Selected Oral Antihypertensives

Drug Category	Onset of Action (mins)	Peak Effect (hrs)	Duration (hrs)
Angiotensin-converting enzyme inhibitors			
Captopril	15	1.0–1.5	Dose related
Enalapril	60	4–8	12–24
Calcium channel blockers			
Diltiazem	30–60	2–3	8–12
Nifedipine (oral)	10–20	30	8
Nifedipine (sublingual)	1–5	—	—
Nifedipine (long acting)	—	5–6	24
Verapamil	30	1–2	6–8
Beta-adrenergic antagonists			
Atenolol	60	2–4	24
Propranolol	60–120	1–3	6–12
Labetalol	20–120	1–4	8–24
Vasodilators			
Hydralazine	20–30	1–2	2–4
Minoxidil	30	2–8	Up to 5 days

Approach to Therapy

Because patients with hypertension are often asymptomatic, patients and families must understand the importance of prolonged BP reduction. Constant attention to dietary factors and daily use of medications in children and adolescents who otherwise feel well, creates a setting for poor compliance. Therefore, ongoing education regarding the risks of sustained hypertension are an essential part of therapy. Patients and families should understand that, in the absence of acute hypertensive episodes, long-term BP reduction is worthwhile in preventing or delaying cardiovascular and other end-organ damage that develops over decades. It is likewise the physician's responsibility to select therapies that maximize the effects of BP reduction. For example, reduction of left ventricular hypertrophy, alterations of metabolic parameters (such as cholesterol and lipid profiles, and glucose metabolism), and reduction of the risk for adverse cardiac events should all be considered when forming a treatment plan. The suggestion for increasing compliance with nonpharmacologic therapies discussed in Chapter 5 may be equally applied to those patients receiving antihypertensive medications.

TABLE 6.27
Comparison of Potential First-Line Medications Used in the Treatment
of Hypertension

	Angiotensin-Converting Enzyme Inhibitors	Calcium Channel Blockers	Beta Blockers	Diuretics
Lipid metabolism	0	+	−	−
Glucose metabolism	0	0	−	−
Left ventricular hypertrophy	+	+	0	−
Exercise tolerance	0	0	−	0
Electrolytes	0	0	0	−

+ = favorable effect; − = unfavorable effect; 0 = neutral or unknown effect.

Recommended Treatment for Specific Causes of Hypertension

Essential Hypertension

When compared with adults, hypertensive children are more likely to have a specific cause of hypertension. Nevertheless, the majority of hypertensive children and adolescents have no identifiable cause and are considered to have essential hypertension. Treatment of mild hypertension in adults is recommended and is beneficial in preventing subsequent atherosclerotic disease and end-organ damage. Deciding to initiate therapy in children is more controversial, particularly in the absence of convincing evidence that hypertensive children become hypertensive adults. BP lability is common, and new technologies for ambulatory BP monitoring may define children with significant BP elevations. However, standardized data are limited and prospective studies are needed. At present, antihypertensive therapy in children with essential hypertension should be conservative. It should attempt to reduce BP and at the same time minimize adverse metabolic effects (e.g., hyperlipidemia, electrolyte abnormalities, glucose intolerance) (Table 6.27), unpleasant side effects (e.g., sedation, behavioral changes), and the psychosocial stigma of being labeled with a lifelong disease.

Figures 6.2 and 6.3 list approaches to the treatment of a child with essential hypertension. Hypertension may not persist into adulthood, and it may be possible to discontinue medications. While the role of ambulatory BP monitoring is not currently well defined, it may become a useful tool in deciding which children are candidates for medications.

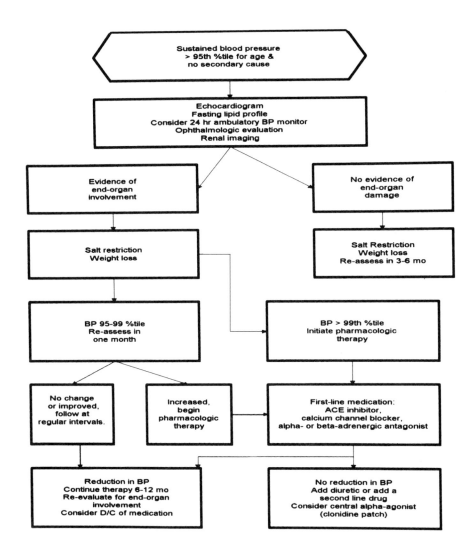

FIGURE 6.2. Treatment of essential hypertension in children and adolescents.

Hypertensive Emergencies

Patients presenting with BP greater than 30% for age require immediate attention [30]. For purposes of treatment, it is useful to consider two situations: (1) hypertensive emergencies—situations in which life- or organ-threatening damage will occur if BP is not reduced immediately, and (2) hypertensive urgencies—situations in which the possibility exists for progression to a hypertensive emergency. It is important to recognize that the absolute value of BP may not indicate the severity of

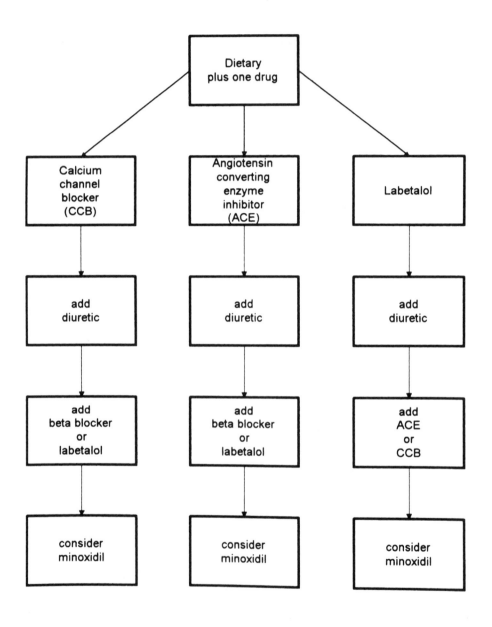

FIGURE 6.3. Specific treatment pathways for essential hypertension.

TABLE 6.28
Hypertensive Emergencies

Hypertensive encephalopathy
Hypertension associated with:
  Acute heart failure
  Pulmonary edema
  Acute renal failure
  Stroke
  Head trauma
  Myocardial infarction
Adrenergic crisis
Dissecting aortic aneurysm
Eclampsia
Malignant hypertension

Source: LG Feld, JE Springate. Hypertension in children. Curr Probl Pediatr 1988;18:319.

BP elevation for a particular patient. Children with nearly "normal" BP for age may develop symptoms of encephalopathy resulting from a significant elevation from their baseline pressures. Rapid falls in BP can result in hypoperfusion of vital organs and iatrogenic morbidity. The distinction between emergencies and urgencies differentiates those patients in whom the benefits of rapid reduction in BP justifies the risks, from those whose BP may be reduced in a stepwise, controlled manner.

Hypertensive emergencies require rapid reduction of BP (usually within 1 hour) to prevent loss of life or vital organ function. Situations include hypertensive encephalopathy (headache, altered mental status, visual impairment, seizures, focal neurologic deficits), malignant hypertension, hypertension associated with acute heart failure, pulmonary edema, acute renal failure, stroke, head trauma, myocardial infarction, adrenergic crisis, dissecting aortic aneurysm, and eclampsia (Table 6.28).

While emergency therapy should include searching for a treatable cause, immediate antihypertensive treatment should not be delayed. Currently available medications for hypertensive emergencies act regardless of the etiology and permit stabilization until a more complete evaluation can proceed. An algorithm for treatment of hypertensive emergencies is shown in Figure 6.4. In addition to the recommendations in the figure, to minimize fluid and salt retention diuretics are indicated in either states of fluid overload or with prolonged use of vasodilators. Beta blockers, while not efficacious in acute BP reduction, may be needed to minimize reflex tachycardia. The goal of emergency therapy for hypertension is a 10–25% reduction in BP in the first hour of therapy. Figure 6.5 provides recommended medications for specific causes of hypertensive emergencies.

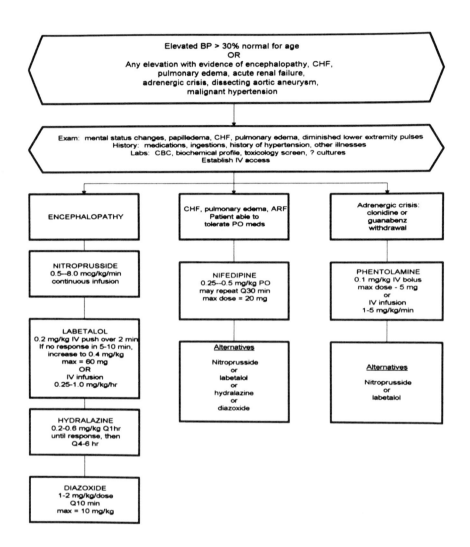

FIGURE 6.4. Treatment of hypertensive emergencies.

Hypertensive urgencies, such as perioperative hypertension and acute increases in BP, that are asymptomatic at presentation permit more conservative reductions in BP, usually over a 24-hour period. In most cases, this can be accomplished with the medications listed in Figure 6.3, although nitroprusside and diazoxide are not indicated. Useful oral drugs include nifedipine, captopril, labetalol, and hydralazine. The availability of both intravenous and oral forms of labetalol and hydralazine is helpful in patients initially unable to tolerate oral medications. Diuretics should be

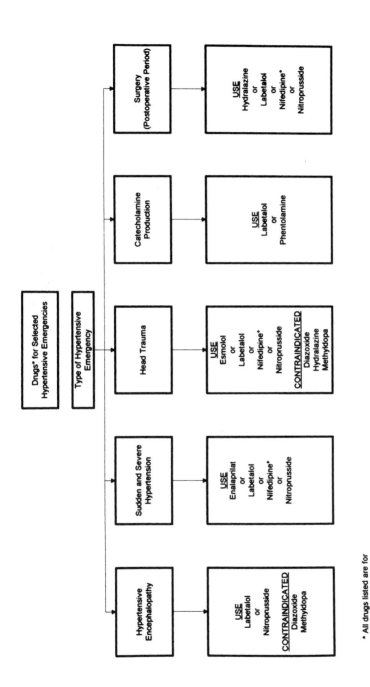

FIGURE 6.5. Recommended medications for specific causes of hypertensive emergencies.

considered as adjunctive therapy in conditions of fluid overload. Patients should be monitored closely for progression to symptomatic hypertension.

Diabetes Mellitus

The frequent occurrence of hypertension in patients with diabetes mellitus significantly increases their risk of cardiac disease, stroke, peripheral vascular disease, retinopathy, and nephropathy [73]. Detection and early treatment of hypertension in diabetic patients can slow the progression of renal and eye disease and lower the incidence of myocardial infarction and stroke. Commonly used in treatment of essential hypertension, high-dosage thiazide diuretics and beta blockers are not indicated as first-line drugs in the therapy of diabetic hypertension. Adverse effects on lipid and glucose metabolism limit their usefulness. Low-dosage thiazide diuretics may be used in combination with ACE inhibitors or CCBs. ACE inhibitors, in addition to their antihypertensive effect, may favorably impact glomerular hemodynamics, thus slowing the progression of diabetic nephropathy [74]. CCBs may also confer renal benefits in addition to their antihypertensive effects [75]. Neither CCBs nor ACE inhibitors adversely effect lipid or glucose metabolism, and they are both recommended as first-line therapy in diabetics. Alpha$_1$-adrenergic blockers are also very effective as a second-line therapy, although orthostatic hypotension may be a problem in patients with diabetes. Alpha and beta blockers, centrally acting alpha$_2$-agonists, and sympatholytic agents should be used with caution. The recommended sequence of therapy is as follows: (1) ACE inhibitors; (2) low-dosage hydrochlorothiazide (25 mg/day); and (3) alpha-adrenergic receptors antagonists or CCBs.

Acute Renal Failure

The hypertension of acute renal failure represents primarily a state of volume overload with relative renal hypoperfusion. Severe hypertension is discussed in the section on hypertensive emergencies. Mild to moderate hypertension in acute renal failure often responds to diuretics and fluid restriction. When the GFR is less than 10 ml/min/1.73 m^2, diuretic efficacy is limited. Use of ACE inhibitors is contraindicated. CCBs and beta blockers are effective, but in refractory cases dialysis may be required to restore euvolemia.

Neonatal Hypertension

The majority of healthy, full-term infants do not have significant hypertension, and there are no recommendations for routine BP monitoring in the first year of life. However, premature infants, ill infants, and those with a family history of congenitally transmitted renal or heart diseases should be monitored. Table 3.3 in Chapter 3 lists causes of neonatal hypertension.

TABLE 6.29
Pharmacologic Therapy of Neonatal Hypertension

Drug	Dosing
Captopril	0.05–0.5 mg/kg/day PO divided q6–8h
Enalaprilat	5–10 µg/kg/dose q8–24h
Hydralazine	Hypertensive crisis: 0.1–0.5 mg/kg/dose IM/IV q4–6h prn Chronic hypertension: 0.5–5.0 mg/kg/day PO divided q6–12h
Chlorothiazide	20–30 mg/kg/day PO divided q12h
Hydrochlorothiazide	2–3 mg/kg/day PO divided q12h
Furosemide	1–4 mg/kg/dose IV/PO q6–8h
Propranolol	0.5–2.0 mg/kg/day PO divided q6–12h
Nitroprusside	0.5–8.0 µg/kg/min continuous IV infusion
Diazoxide	1–2 mg/kg/dose IV q10 mins up to 10 mg/kg/day

Essential hypertension is an uncommon diagnosis in neonates: A secondary cause should always be sought. Pharmacologic therapy is effective in reducing BP and is often necessary only until a cause can be found and treated. Medications used in neonatal hypertension are listed in Table 6.29.

Chronic Renal Failure

Systemic hypertension is one of the major problems assoicated with chronic renal disease in infants and children. In most cases of chronic renal insufficiency, the treatment of systemic hypertension comprises a significant amount of the effort in both inpatient and outpatient settings. Based on studies in adults and in animal models of experimental kidney disease, nephrologists agree that effective control of blood pressure delays can prevent the progression of chronic renal failure. With this information, two key management questions emerge: (1) Does the selected antihypertensive drug influence the kidney response? and (2) What is the optimum blood pressure values for a child with kidney disease? [76].

The prevalence of hypertension varies with the cause of kidney failure. In our experience, prevalence of systemic hypertension in patients with established, progressive renal disease (reduction in GFR <50 ml/minute/1.73m^2) can be categorized as (1) frequent (>50%), (2) common (10–50%), and (3) unusual (<10%) (Table 6.30). As a general rule, hypertension is infrequent in congenital renal disease and is a universal finding in primary glomerular disease and kidney injury secondary to systemic disease.

The diurnal variation in systemic BP is reversed in patients with chronic renal insufficiency [77]. In such cases, the expected drop in systemic BP at night (nocturnal hypotension) is lost. Nighttime BPs exceed daytime values in the majority of pediatric patients with kidney disease

TABLE 6.30
Prevalence Rates of Systemic Hypertension in Patients with Established
Progressive Renal Failure

Frequent
　Focal segmental glomerulosclerosis
　Chronic glomerulonephritis
　Mesangial proliferative glomerulonephritis
　Diabetic nephropathy
　Systemic lupus erythematosus (sclerosing, diffuse proliferative)
　Systemic vasculitis (Wegener's granulomatosis, Henoch-Schönlein purpura,
　　polyarteritis nodosa, etc)
　Hemolytic-uremic syndrome
　Advanced reflux nephropathy
　Rapidly progressive glomerulonephritis
　Polycystic kidney disease
　Glomerulocystic disease
Common
　IgA nephropathy (uncommon unless with significant proteinuria or impaired
　　renal function)
　Membranoproliferative glomerulonephritis (especially with steroid treatment)
　HIV-associated nephropathy
Unusual
　Interstitial nephritis
　Obstructive uropathy
　Sickle cell nephropathy
　Alport's syndrome
　Medullary cystic disease
　Renal hypoplasia/dysplasia
　Membranous nephropathy

Source: Reproduced with permission from LG Feld, E Lieberman, SA Mendoza, JE
Springate. Management of hypertension in the child with chronic renal failure. J Pediatr
1996;129(Suppl):S18.

[78]. This high prevalence of moderate to severe hypertension during the
night requires additional antihypertensive therapy.

Regardless of the etiology of chronic renal failure, hypertension accelerates the decline in the glomerular filtration rate. Increased systemic BP
can damage the kidney by stimulating myointimal hyperplasia and hypertrophy of renal arterioles and by increasing glomerular capillary (intrarenal)
hydrostatic pressure [79]. The first mechanism causes hypertensive
microangiopathy with subsequent ischemia and death of nephrons.
Through direct barotrauma to the glomerulus, the second mechanism causes albuminuria, mesangial expansion, and eventual glomerular sclerosis.

In patients with chronic renal disease, BP should be gradually reduced
to prevent decreased renal perfusion and reduction in renal function [80].

TABLE 6.31
Selected Antihypertensive Drugs for Patients with Chronic Renal Failure

Drug	Formulation	Dose (oral)	Adjustment in Chronic Renal Failure	Effect on Renin
Diuretics				Increase
Chlorothiazide	250- and 500-mg tablets, 250 mg/5 ml	5–10 mg/kg/dose bid	Thiazides not effective at glomerular filtration rate (GFR)	
Hydrochloro-thiazide	25-, 50-, and 100-mg tablets, 50 mg/5 ml; 100 mg/ml	0.5–2.0 mg/kg/dose qd or bid	<30–40 ml/min/1.73 m^2	
Furosemide	20-, 40-, and 80-mg tablets, 10 mg/ml	0.5–4.0 mg/kg/dose qd or bid	None	
Bumetanide	0.5-, 1-, and 2-mg tablets	0.01–0.03 mg/dose qd	Unknown	
Metolazone	2.5-, 5-, and 10-mg tablets, 0.1 mg/ml	0.2 mg/kg/dose qd or bid	Unknown	
Beta blockers				Decrease
Acebutolol	200- and 400-mg tablets	200–800 mg qd (adults)	Decrease dose	
Atenolol	25-, 50-, and 100-mg tablets	50–100 mg (adults)	Decrease 50% at GFR <50 ml/min/1.73 m^2, give qod GFR <10 ml/min/1.73 m^2	
Labetalol	100-, 200-, and 300-mg tablets	50–100 mg bid (>10 yrs of age)	None	
Metoprolol	50- and 100-mg tablets	100–200 mg qd or bid (adults)	None	
Propranolol	10-, 20-, 40-, 60-, and 80-mg tablets 20, 40, and 80 mg/ml	0.5–1.0 mg/dose bid	None	
Vasodilators				Increase
Hydralazine	10-, 25-, 50-, and 100-mg tablets 0.2 mg/ml	0.5–2.0 mg/kg/dose bid or qid	None	
Minoxidil	2.5- and 10-mg tablets	0.1–0.5 mg/kg/dose bid to qd	None	

TABLE 6.31. *(continued)*

Drug	Formulation	Dose (oral)	Adjustment in Chronic Renal Failure	Effect on Renin
Central sympatholytic				Decrease
Clonidine	0.1-, 0.2-, and 0.3-mg tablets or patch	0.05–0.30 mg/ dose bid or tid	None	
Angiotensin-converting enzyme inhibitors				Increase
			Caution with all ACE inhibitors when GFR <50 ml/min/1.73 m²	
Captopril	12.5-, 25-, 50-, and 100-mg tablets	0.5–2.0 mg/ kg/day bid		
Enalapril	2.5-. 5-, 10-, and 20-mg tablets	0.15 mg/kg/day bid		
Fosinopril	10- and 20-mg tablets	5–20 mg qd (adults)		
Lisinopril	2.5-, 5-, 10-, 20-, and 40-mg tablets	2.5–20.0 mg/day bid or qd (adults)		
Calcium channel blockers				None
Nifedipine	10- and 20-mg caplets 30-, 60-, and 90-mg sustained release	0.25–2.0 mg/ kg/dose bid to qid sustained release qd or bid	May need to limit dose	
Diltiazem	30-, 60-, 90-, 120-mg tablets 120-, 180-, 240-, and 300- mg caplets	0.40–1.25 mg/ kg/dose qid sustained release qd to bid	Unknown	
Verapamil	120-, 180-, and 240-mg tablets	4–10 mg/kg/ day tid	With caution	

Source: Reproduced with permission from LG Feld, E Lieberman, SA Mendoza, JE Springate. Management of hypertension in the child with chronic renal failure. J Pediatr 1996;129(Suppl):S18.

of hypertension can lead to a hypertensive emergency resulting in permanent neurologic damage. With aggressive control of hypertension in children with moderate to severe renal insufficiency, the rate of progression to end-stage renal disease may be delayed and cardiovascular damage prevented.

Pheochromocytoma

Treatment pathways of hypertensive crisis secondary to pheochromocytoma are listed in Figure 6.4. Chronic therapy often requires the use of medications that are not routinely used in the treatment of other forms of hypertension. Such medications are discussed briefly here.

Phenoxybenzamine is an orally available alpha-adrenergic antagonist. It reduces BP and symptoms of excessive diaphoresis in patients with pheochromocytoma. It does not block beta-adrenergic receptors. Because of significant effects of alpha blockade (i.e., tachycardia, postural hypotension, inhibition of ejaculation, nasal congestion, miosis, gastrointestinal irritation, drowsiness, and fatigue), it is not useful in treating other forms of hypertension. Dosage should begin at 2.5 mg twice daily and be increased slowly (allow 4–7 days for dosages to take effect) to maximize BP response or until other effects are intolerable. The maximum dosage is 40–100 mg/day in adolescents and older children and 20–25 mg/day in younger children. Concomitant use of a beta blocker is often required to control tachycardia.

Metyrosine (Demser) inhibits catecholamine synthesis. It inhibits tyrosine hydroxylase, preventing the conversion of tyrosine to dihydroxyphenylalanine (dopa). Metyrosine is indicated in patients with pheochromocytoma for the following: (1) preoperative preparation for surgery, (2) management of pheochromocytoma when surgery is contraindicated, and (3) chronic treatment of malignant pheochromocytoma. Adverse effects include sedation, extrapyramidal signs (i.e., drooling, speech difficulty, tremor, trismus), anxiety, depression, hallucinations, confusion, diarrhea, crystalluria (metyrosine crystalluria), and ejaculatory difficulty, as well as eosinophilia, thrombocytopenia, anemia, thrombocytosis, elevated serum glutamic-osaloacetic transaminase (SGOT) levels, peripheral edema, and anaphylactic reactions. Dosage is 25–50 mg/kg/day in four divided doses, and may be increased daily to a maximum dosage of 4 g/day in adults. Pediatric experience is limited, and no maximum daily dosage is reported for children under 12 years of age.

References

1. Sinaiko AR. Pharmacologic management of childhood hypertension. Pediatr Clin North Am 1993;40:195.

2. Jung FF, Ingelfinger JR. Hypertension in childhood and adolescence. Pediatr Rev 1993;14:169.

3. Waeber B, Nussberger J, Brunner H. Angiotensin Converting–Enzyme Inhibitors in Hypertension. In JH Laragh, BM Brenner (eds), Hypertension: Pathophysiology, Diagnosis, and Management. New York: Raven, 1990;2209.

4. Kostis JB. Angiotensin converting enzyme inhibitors: emerging differences and new compounds. Am J Hypertens 1989;2:57.

5. Mirkin BL, Newman TJ. Efficacy and safety of captopril in the treatment of severe childhood hypertension: report of the international collaborative study group. Pediatrics 1985;75:1091.

6. Sinaiko AR, Kashtan CE, Mirkin BL. Antihypertensive drug therapy with captopril in children and adolescents. Clin Exp Theory Practice 1986;8:829.

7. Bendig L, Temesvari A. Indications and effects of captopril therapy in childhood. Acta Physiol Hung 1988;72:121.

8. Schneeweiss A. Cardiovascular drugs in children II: angiotensin converting enzyme inhibitors in pediatrics. Pediatr Cardiol 1990;11:199.

9. O'Dea RF, Mirkin BL, Alward CT, Sinaiko AR. Treatment of neonatal hypertension with captopril. J Pediatr 1988;113:403.

10. Wells TG, Bunchman TE, Kearns GL. Treatment of neonatal hypertension with enalaprilat. J Pediatr 1990;117:664.

11. Shahar E, Sagy M, Koren G, Barzilay Z. Calcium blocking agents in pediatric emergency care. Pediatr Emerg Care 1990;6:52.

12. Barst RJ, Stalcup SA, Steeg CN, et al. Relation of arachidonate metabolites to abnormal control of the pulmonary circulation in a child. Am Rev Respir Dis 1985;13:171.

13. Bertorini TE, Palmieri GMA, Griffin JW, et al. Effect of chronic treatment with the calcium antagonist diltiazem in Duchenne muscular dystrophy. Neurology 1988;38:609.

14. Lepoittevin L, Pezard P, Victor J, Granry JC. Treatment of neonatal supraventricular tachycardia with injectable diltiazem. Presse Med 1989;18:82.

15. Foresi A, Corbo GM, Ciappi G, et al. Effect of two doses of inhaled diltiazem on exercise-induced asthma. Respiration 1987;51:241.

16. Loutzenhiser R, Epstein M. Calcium antagonists and the kidney. Am J Hypertens 1989;2:1545.

17. Reams GP, Bauer JH. Effects of calcium antagonists on the hypertensive kidney. Cardiovasc Drugs Ther 1990;4:1331.

18. Benstein JA, Dworkin LD. Renal vascular effects of calcium channel blockers in hypertension. Am J Hypertens 1990;3:305.

19. Fuberg CD, Psaty BM, Meyer JV. Nifedipine. Dose-related increase in mortality in patients with coronary heart disease. Circulation 1995;92:1326.

20. Dilmen U, Caglar K, Senses A, Kinik E. Nifedipine in hypertensive emergencies of children. Am J Dis Child 1983;137:1162.

21. Roth B, Herkenrath P, Krebber J, Abu-Chaaban M. Nifedipine in hypertensive crises of infants and children. Clin Exp Theory Practice 1986;A8:871.

22. Rascher W, Bonzel KE, Ruder H, et al. Blood pressure and hormonal responses to sublingual nifedipine in acute childhood hypertension. Clin Exp Theory Practice 1986;A8:859.

23. Lopez-Herce J, Albajara L, Cagigas P, et al. Treatment of hypertensive crisis in children with nifedipine. Intensive Care Med 1988;14:519.

24. Ogborn MR, Crocker JFS, Grimm PC. Nifedipine, verapamil, and cyclosporin A pharmacokinetics in children. Pediatr Nephrol 1989;3:314.

25. Bolli P, Fernandez PG, Buhler F. Beta-Blockers in the Treatment of Hypertension. In JH Laragh, BM Brenner (eds), Hypertension: Pathophysiology, Diagnosis, and Management. New York: Raven, 1990;2181.

26. Goldberg M, Fenster PE. Clinical significance of intrinsic sympathomimetic activity of beta blockers. Drug Therapy 1991;June:35.

27. Kornbluth A, Frishman WH, Ackerman M. Beta adrenergic blockade in children. Cardiol Clin North Am 1987;5:629.

28. Mongeau J, Biron P, Pichardo LM. Propranolol Efficacy in Adolescent Essential Hypertension. In MI New, LS Levine (eds), Juvenile Hypertension. New York: Raven, 1977;219.

29. Mirkin BL, Sinaiko A. Clinical Pharmacology and Therapeutic Utilization of Antihypertensive Agents in Children. In MI New, LS Levine (eds), Juvenile Hypertension. New York: Raven, 1977;195.

30. Feld LG, Springate JE. Hypertension in children. Curr Probl Pediatr 1988;18:319.

31. Hanna JD, Chan JCM, Gill JR. Hypertension and the kidney. J Pediatr 1991;118:327.

32. Thompson WG. Review: an assault on old friends: thiazide diuretics under siege. Am J Med Sci 1990;300:152.

33. Parijs J, Joosens JV, Van der Linden L, et al. Moderate sodium restriction and diuretics in the treatment of hypertension. Am Heart J 1973;85:22.

34. Ram CVS, Garrett BN, Kaplan NM. Moderate sodium restriction and various diuretics in the treatment of hypertension. Arch Intern Med 1981;141:1015.

35. Pecker MS. Pathophysiologic Effects and Strategies for Long-Term Diuretic Treatment of Hypertension. In JH Laragh, BM Brenner (eds), Hypertension: Pathophysiology, Diagnosis, and Management. New York: Raven, 1990;2143.

36. Haddy FJ, Pamnani MB, Swindall BT, et al. Sodium channel blockers are vasodilators as well as natriuretic and diuretic agents. Hypertension 1985;7(Suppl I):121.

37. Bennett WM, McDonald WJ, Kuehnel E, et al. Do diuretics have antihypertensive properties independent of natriuresis? Clin Pharmacol Ther 1977;22:499.

38. Chemtob S, Kaplan BS, Sherbotie JR, Aranda JV. Pharmacology of diuretics in the newborn. Pediatr Clin North Am 1989;36:1231.

39. Wahling TM, Thompson TR, Sinaiko AR. Drug use in the newborn: effects on the kidney. Clin Perinatol 1992;19:251.

40. Wells TG. The pharmacology and therapeutics of diuretics in the pediatric patient. Pediatr Clin North Am 1990;37:463.

41. Prandota J, Pruitt AW. Furosemide binding to human albumin and plasma of nephrotic children. Clin Pharmacol Ther 1975;17:159.
42. Brummett RE, Bendrick T, Himes D. Comparative ototoxicity of bumetanide and furosemide when used in combination with kanamycin. J Clin Pharmacol 1981;21:628.
43. Lynn AM, Redding GJ, Morray JP. Isolated deafness following recovery from neurologic injury and adult respiratory distress syndrome: a sequelae of intercurrent aminoglycoside and diuretic use. Am J Dis Child 1985;139:464.
44. Robinson F, Benjamin N. Vasodilators. In JH Laragh, BM Brenner (eds), Hypertension: Pathophysiology, Diagnosis, and Management. New York: Raven, 1990;2263.
45. Jacobs M. Mechanism of action of hydralazine on vascular smooth muscle. Biochem Pharmacol 1984;33:2915.
46. Spokas EG, Folco G, Quilley J, et al. Endothelial mechanism in the vascular action of hydralazine. Hypertension 1983;5(Suppl I):107.
47. Martin GR, Chauvin L, Short BL. Effects of hydralazine on cardiac performance in infants receiving extracorporeal membrane oxygenation. J Pediatr 1991;118:944.
48. Sofer S, Gueron M. Vasodilators and hypertensive encephalopathy following scorpion envenomation in children. Chest 1990;97:118.
49. Adelman RD, Merten D, Vogel J, et al. Nonsurgical treatment of renovascular hypertension in the neonate. Pediatrics 1978;62:71.
50. Irias JJ. Hydralazine-induced lupus erythematosus–like syndrome. Am J Dis Child 1975;129:862.
51. Yemini M, Shoham Z, Dgani R, Lancet M. Lupus-like syndrome in a mother and newborn following administration of hydralazine: a case report. Eur J Obstet Gynecol Reprod Biol 1989;30:193.
52. Meisheri KD, Cipkus LA. Minoxidil sulfate acts as a K^+-channel agonist to produce vasodilation [abstract]. Fed Proc 1987;46:1383.
53. Puri HC, Maltz HE, Kaiser BA, Potter DE. Severe hypertension in children with renal disease: treatment with minoxidil. Am J Kidney Dis 1983;3:71.
54. Sinaiko AR, O'Dea RF, Mirkin BL. Clinical response of hypertensive children to long-term minoxidil therapy. J Cardiovasc Pharmacol 1980;2(Suppl 2):181.
55. Pennisi AJ, Takahashi M, Bernstein BH, Singsen BH. Minoxidil therapy in children with severe hypertension. J Pediatr 1977;90:813.
56. Bunchman TE, Lynch RE, Wood EG. Intravenously administered labetalol for treatment of hypertension in children. J Pediatr 1992;120:140.
57. Miller RR, Vismara LA, Williams DO, et al. Pharmacological mechanisms for left ventricular unloading in clinical congestive heart failure. Differential effects of nitroprusside, phentolamine, and nitroglycerine on cardiac function and peripheral circulation. Circ Res 1976;39:127.
58. Palmer RMJ, Ferrige AC, Moncada S. Nitric oxide accounts for the biological activity of endothelium-derived relaxing factor. Nature 1987;327:524.
59. Snyder SH, Bredt DS. Biological roles of nitric oxide. Sci Am 1992;266:68.

60. Ignarro LJ, Lippton H, Edwards JC. Mechanism of vascular smooth muscle relaxation by organic nitrates, nitrites, nitroprusside, and nitric oxide: evidence for the involvement of S-nitrothiols as active intermediates. J Pharmacol Exp Ther 1991;218:739.

61. Parmer RJ, O'Connor DT. Central Sympthetic Agents in the Treatment of Hypertension. In WM Bennett, DA McCarron, BM Brenner, JH Stein (eds), Contemporary Issues in Nephrology #17: Pharmacotherapy of Renal Disease and Hypertension. New York: Churchill Livingstone, 1987;255.

62. Shapiro AP, Schwartz GE, Ferguson DC, et al. Behavioral methods in the treatment of hypertension. A review of their clinical status. Ann Intern Med 1977;86:626.

63. Oster JR, Epstein M. Use of centrally acting sympatholytic agents in the management of hypertension. Arch Intern Med 1991;151:1638.

64. Yamori Y, Nara Y, Mano M, Horie R. Sympathetic factors in the cardiovascular complications of hypertension: evidence in genetic models for hypertension, stroke, and atherosclerosis. J Hypertens 1985;3(Suppl 4):35.

65. Weber MA, Graettinger WF, Cheung DG. Centrally Acting Sympathetic Inhibitors. In JH Laragh, BM Brenner (eds), Hypertension: Pathophysiology, Diagnosis, and Management. New York: Raven, 1990;2251.

66. Comings DE, Comings BG, Tacket T, Li SZ. The clonidine patch and behavior problems. J Am Acad Child Adolesc Psychiatry 1990;29:667.

67. Huisjes HJ, Hadders-Algra M, Towen BC. Is clonidine a behavioral teratogen in the human? Early Hum Devel 1986;14:43.

68. Fiser DH, Moss MM, Walker W. Critical care for clonidine poisoning in toddlers. Crit Care Med 1990;18:1124.

69. Dawson PM, Vander Zanden JA, Werkman SL, et al. Cardiac dysrhythmia with use of clonidine in explosive disorder. Drug Intelligence and Clinical Pharmacy 1989;23:465.

70. Artman M, Boerth RC. Clonidine poisoning: a complex problem. Am J Dis Child 1983;137:171.

71. Kaplan NM. Effects of guanabenz on plasma lipid levels in hypertensive patients. J Cardiovasc Pharmacol 1984;6:841.

72. Pool JL, Taylor AA, Nelson EB. Review of the effects of doxazosin, a new selective alpha-1 adrenergic inhibitor, on lipoproteins in patients with essential hypertension. Am J Med 1989;87(Suppl 2A):57.

73. Epstein M, Sowers JR. Diabetes mellitus and hypertension. Hypertension 1992;19:403.

74. Zatz R, Dunn BR, Meyer TW, et al. Prevention of diabetic glomerulopathy by pharmacological amelioration of glomerular capillary hypertension. J Clin Invest 1986;77:1925.

75. Epstein M. Calcium antagonists and diabetic nephropathy. Arch Intern Med 1991;151:2361.

76. Hollenberg NK. Does antihypertensive therapy retard progression of renal disease? Choices Cardiol 1990;5:8.

77. Portman RJ, Yetman RJ. Clinical uses of ambulatory blood pressure monitoring. Pediatr Nephrol 1994;8:367.
78. Rodriquez OJ, Yetman RJ, West MS, Portman RJ. Unexpected diagnosis of nocturnal hypertension in pediatric renal patients by the ambulatory blood pressure monitor. Pediatr Res 1991;29:351.
79. Buckalew VM. Pathophysiology of progressive renal failure. South Med J 1994;87:1028.
80. Feld LG, Lieberman E, Mendoza SA, Springate JE. Management of hypertension in the child with chronic renal failure. J Pediatr 1996;129(Suppl):S18.

CHAPTER 7

Special Considerations in Pediatric Hypertension

James E. Springate

Obesity and Hypertension

The 1987 Task Force Report on Pediatric Hypertension recommends that obesity-associated hypertension be considered in all children who appear obese with blood pressures (BPs) and weights above the ninetieth percentile for age and sex [1]. Numerous studies have demonstrated that adults, adolescents, and children with otherwise unexplained high BP are often overweight and that obesity is an important risk factor for future hypertension [2]. In addition, weight reduction is a successful treatment for hypertension in many obese patients. Epidemiologic research suggests that approximately 45% of young people with high BP who are seen by primary care providers are also overweight [3]. In a study comparing data from 1963 to 1965 with data from 1976 to 1980, Gortmaker and colleagues [4] found a 54% increase in the prevalence of obesity and a 98% increase in severe obesity in children 6–11 years old. A similar trend was also found in adolescents: Their prevalence of obesity and severe obesity increased by 39% and 64%, respectively. These investigators also noted a 13–16% increase in the incidence of obesity-associated hypertension during the period of the study. These alarming statistics clearly indicate that greater attention to the treatment and prevention of pediatric obesity is needed.

The pathogenesis of obesity-related hypertension has not been clearly defined. Current research suggests that it relates to dysfunctional regulation of vascular tone, intravascular volume, or both [5, 6]. As body fat increases, there is more tissue to perfuse, and cardiac output rises. Expansion of circulating blood volume appears to be primarily responsible for augmenting cardiac output in obesity. Because arterial pressure is proportional to cardiac output and systemic vascular resistance, the only way to maintain normal BP in the face of increasing cardiac output is to lower vascular resistance. Overweight subjects with normal BPs have an elevated cardiac output and blood volume and a decreased systemic vascular resistance. However, vascular resistance in obese hypertensive patients is typically either unexpectedly normal or increased. To date, no specific mechanism has been found to explain the failure of vascular tone to decrease as cardiac output rises in these individuals. Altered sympathetic nervous system activity may play a role in this process [7].

Although some degree of volume expansion is physiologically appropriate in obesity, excessive intravascular volume may also contribute to obesity-associated hypertension. In a study of obese adolescents, Rocchini and colleagues [8] found that salt restriction without weight loss significantly reduced arterial pressure by a mean of 12 mm Hg. This advantageous decline in BP was accompanied by substantial reductions in cardiac output and plasma volume. These latter measurements, however, remained significantly greater than those of nonobese teenagers receiving either high- or low-salt diets. The overly expanded plasma volume and salt-sensitive BP of obese children indicate an abnormality in the renal function that normally adjusts salt and water excretion to achieve normal intravascular volume and BP. Interestingly, subsequent weight loss in the same patients not only normalized BP but also eliminated its sodium sensitivity. These changes were accompanied by correction of increased sympathetic nervous system activity, hyperaldosteronism, and hyperinsulinemia, suggesting that these abnormalities may be involved in obesity-related hypertension.

There has been tremendous interest in the possible role of insulin in producing hypertension associated with obesity. Hyperinsulinemia and insulin resistance are commonly found in overweight individuals [9]. The mechanisms by which these abnormalities may produce high BP were reviewed by DeFronzo and Ferrannini [10]. They are (1) insulin-induced impairment of renal sodium excretion leading to intravascular volume expansion; (2) increased sympathetic nervous system activity produced by excessive insulin, which subsequently causes vasoconstriction, increased cardiac output, and enhanced aldosterone secretion; (3) interference with cell membrane pumps that control responsiveness to various vasoactive substances; and (4) stimulation of vascular and cardiac muscle growth leading to vessel narrowing and cardiac hypertrophy. Although the hyperinsulinemia hypothesis has proved to be a new and exciting aspect of research in hypertension, it is by no means clear that insulin plays a predominant role in BP control during obesity [6].

Clinically, the diagnosis of obesity-related hypertension raises several issues. First, it is extremely important that the appropriate cuff size be

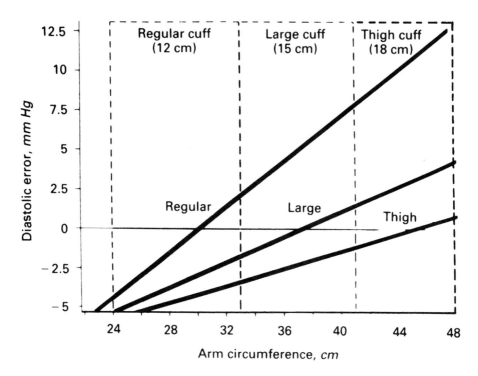

FIGURE 7.1. Relationship between diastolic blood pressure and arm circumference. (Reproduced with permission from LP Dornfield, MH Maxwell, A Waks, M Tuck. Mechanisms of hypertension in obesity. Used with permission from Kidney International, volume 32, page S254, 1987.)

used in measurement. Maxwell and colleagues [11] analyzed 84,000 BP measurements in 1,240 obese individuals using different cuff sizes. They found large errors in BP readings when inappropriately small cuffs were used. Their data relating mid-upper arm circumference, cuff size, and BP measurements allow selection of the best cuff size for determining BP in specific patients (Figure 7.1).

Second, obesity, or excessive fatness, must be defined. Sophisticated measurements of adiposity, such as hydrometry, hydrodensitometry, ^{40}K spectrometry, and total-body electrical conductivity, are technically difficult and impractical [12]. Although skinfold thickness is often used as a measure of fatness in children, there are problems with this technique. Skinfold thickness is usually obtained at only one or a limited number of sites. Site-specific subcutaneous fat deposits vary widely in relation to age, sex, race, and body habitus and may not accurately reflect total body fat [13]. In addition, this technique is often unreliable because of interobserver variation and differences in types of calipers [13]. For these reasons, most clinicians continue to rely on growth charts to define obesity. In general, children who weigh 20% or more above the mean weight for their height can be considered obese if inspection confirms that their excessive weight is the result of fat and not lean body mass. This simple calculation not only provides a more objective measure of fatness than visual inspection but also permits an estimate of "ideal" or "target" weight for use in planning treatment. The body mass or Quelelet index (weight per height^2) has been recommended as a simple, reasonably accurate measure of obesity in adults by the National Institutes of Health Panel on Obesity [14]. Standardized percentile curves of body mass index have been developed for children and adolescents [13]. Their generalized use may facilitate patient care and research in pediatric obesity.

The final clinical issue raised by obesity-related hypertension is confirmation of the diagnosis. This can only be accomplished by documenting a reduction of BP with weight loss. Treatment of childhood obesity is difficult and optimally involves a program of diet, exercise, and other life-style changes with support from medical professionals, nutritionists, and family members [15]. Unfortunately, this treatment is often unsuccessful. The diagnosis of obesity-associated hypertension then becomes a matter of clinical judgment and some degree of uncertainty. In general, as the 1987 Task Force Report notes, "obese children are unlikely to have a cause for their high BP other than their excessive ponderosity" [1]. Nevertheless, obese hypertensive children with severely high BP or with any degree of hypertension refractory to weight reduction should receive the same evaluation and management as their nonobese counterparts. Particular attention should be paid to excluding unusual causes of secondary hypertension associated with obesity, such as Cushing's syndrome and sleep apnea [16]. Sleep apnea is receiving increased attention as a potential cause of systemic hypertension to the extent that inquiries about snoring, hypersomnolence, and morning tiredness should be a routine part of the evaluation of hypertensive patients [17]. Overweight children and their families should also be aware that the persistence of obesity and hypertension into adulthood dramatically increases the risk of heart disease [2].

Drugs Exacerbating Hypertension

A number of medications are associated with high BP. Table 4.2 lists drugs with the potential for increasing BP that might be used in pediatric practice. These prescription and over-the-counter medications are not necessarily contraindicated in hypertensive children, particularly if alternative forms of treatment are not available. However, careful monitoring is clearly advisable, with subsequent modification of treatment if adverse effects arise. This section discusses in detail those drugs with significant hypertensive properties that are commonly encountered in pediatrics.

Phenylpropanolamine is an amphetamine-like alpha$_1$-agonist causing vasoconstriction and increased BP. It was originally synthesized as an intravenous pressor agent but was subsequently marketed as a nasal decongestant and anorectic. Presently, more than 100 products contain phenylpropanolamine, most of these are sold over-the-counter as cough and cold remedies or diet aids. Although the amount of phenylpropanolamine taken by children is unknown, sales of this drug generate more than $200 million dollars in annual revenues [18].

Prospective, well-controlled research in adults on the effects of phenylpropanolamine on BP have shown dramatic increases in BP [19]. In one study, 150 mg (approximately 2 mg/kg) of phenylpropanolamine raised BP to a mean value of 173/103 mm Hg, and 75 mg (approximately 1 mg/kg) raised BP to a mean value of 149/98 mm Hg, both from baseline readings averaging 124/73 mm Hg [20]. The peak effect of phenylpropanolamine on BP occurred about 2–3 hours after ingestion. Similar studies are not available in children or in patients with high BP. Impressed by the hypertensive potential of phenylpropanolamine, Lake and colleagues [18] analyzed all reported adverse drug reactions to this medication. They found 142 cases of adverse reactions to phenylpropanolamine-containing products. Twenty-four percent of these patients were less than 20 years of age, and, as is often the case involving preadolescents, none of the reactions resulted from accidental poisonings. Most adverse reactions (85%) were associated with over-the-counter products. A common presenting feature of most reactions was either severe hypertension or symptoms, such as severe headache, that suggest elevated BP. Many patients developed intracranial hemorrhage or hypertensive encephalopathy. Although the preceding information does not definitively establish the danger of phenylpropanolamine, it clearly indicates that use of products containing this or other adrenergic drugs should be discouraged in hypertensive children. Nasal phenylephrine hydrochloride and oral pseudoephedrine hydrochloride may be the safest of these agents, if required [21, 22]. However, given the questionable value of most cold medicines in children [23], avoiding their use appears the best option.

Sexual activity and pregnancy are becoming increasingly prevalent in adolescent girls. Oral contraceptives are an effective nonsurgical method of contraception and a popular method of birth control among teenagers who practice effective contraception [24]. These medications are also associated with hypertension, with the overall risk for the user being approximately two to three times higher than that of a nonuser. According to one report, combination oral contraceptives cause high BP in about 4–5% of normal women and increase BP in about 9–16% of women with pre-existing hypertension [25]. However, many studies of hypertension and oral contraceptives were performed using dosages of estrogen and progestions that are higher than those currently in use.

Low-dose oral contraceptives (≤35 µg estrogen) are generally prescribed for most healthy young women. If hypertension develops after initiating an oral contraceptive, the medication should be discontinued and nonhormonal forms of contraception initiated. The hypertensive effect of hormonal contraceptives develops within the first 3 months of use and is usually short-lived [24, 25]. Normalization of BP will eliminate the need for a more extensive evaluation. The decision to restart oral contraceptives in this setting should be individualized. If the patient has frequent sexual intercourse and poor compliance with other birth control methods, the clinician may choose to resume hormonal contraception. Progestin-only preparations (e.g.,"mini-pills," DEPO-PROVERA) may be appropriate in these conditions, because they appear to have minimal effects on BP [25]. Hypertension is considered a relative contraindication to hormonal contraception. If the risks of pregnancy clearly outweigh the risks of worsening BP control or other cardiovascular disease risk factors, oral contraceptives can be cautiously prescribed with careful follow-up.

Nonsteroidal anti-inflammatory drugs (NSAIDs) are being used with increasing frequency in pediatrics. These medications have antipyretic, analgesic, and anti-inflammatory properties and are available both by prescription and over-the-counter. NSAIDs can block the action of antihypertensive medications, sometimes producing severe BP elevations [26]. This side effect is often overlooked in the management of hypertensive children.

NSAIDs prevent the synthesis of prostaglandins by inhibiting cyclooxygenase. This enzyme is responsible for transforming arachidonic acid into prostaglandin (PG) G_2 and PGH_2, the common precursors for PG synthesis [27]. The adverse effects of NSAIDs appear to be due to deficient production of vasodilatory prostaglandins, such as prostacyclin and PGE_2 [28]. These substances not only dilate vascular beds but also promote renal sodium excretion; both of these actions favor BP reduction.

NSAIDs do not influence BP in normal individuals [29]. In hypertensive patients, they only modestly raise arterial pressure (up to 10 mm Hg in some studies) [29]. It is only in hypertensive patients receiving antihypertensive drugs that NSAIDs appear to cause substantial elevations in BP [30, 31]. Increases exceeding 40 mm Hg have been documented in some controlled studies, and several cases of hypertensive emergencies coincident with NSAID use have been reported. With the exception of calcium channel blockers, this adverse effect appears to be independent of the type of antihypertensive medication used [26].

The severity of hypertension produced by NSAIDs varies substantially among patients. Some individuals experience no change in BP, while others have massive pressure elevations. Current research suggests that these differences relate, at least in part, to baseline renin-angiotensin system activity. The pressor effect of NSAIDs appears to be most dramatic in low-renin hypertension, although these medications can actually lower BP in highly renin-dependent forms of hypertension such as renal artery stenosis [29]. A potential explanation for this dichotomy may be that prostaglandins can stimulate renal secretion of renin that raises BP through the action of angiotensin II. Inhibition of prostaglandin synthesis by NSAIDs could therefore favorably influence BP control when hyper-reninism is the predominant cause of hypertension. In other situations, loss of the vasodilatory and natriuretic effects of prostaglandins override renin suppression and antagonize the effect of antihypertensive medications. Further research is needed to clarify the influence of renin status on the hypertensive action of NSAIDs before definitive statements regarding their safety in high-renin forms of hypertension can be made.

Although most NSAIDs potentially antagonize the effects of antihypertensive medications, sulindac does not and may be safer to use in hypertensive patients [26, 28]. The reason for this discrepancy is not clear, but it may be due to differences in drug metabolism and sites of action. For example, sulindac sulfide, the active metabolite of sulindac, is inactivated by the kidney; therefore renal cyclo-oxygenase is relatively unaffected by this medication [32]. Continued production of vasodilatory prostaglandins by the kidney might therefore counteract the deleterious effect of NSAIDs on BP control.

Hypertension in Blacks

Adult blacks have a higher incidence of hypertension than whites [33]. In addition, the morbidity and mortality of essential hypertension in the United States is much greater in blacks than in whites, making it a major public health problem [33]. Although a number of studies have shown little or no significant difference in BP values between black and white children, a few have found that elevated BPs are more prevalent among black than white adolescents [34]. One study suggests that these early differences may relate to the fact that blacks tend to be taller, heavier, and more sexually mature than same-aged whites [35]. This section explores potential explanations of the racial differences in both BP and target-organ damage. Treatment of hypertension in black patients will also be discussed.

Physiologic differences in BP control systems exist between black and white children. Blacks exposed to physiologic or psychological stressors experience greater increases in BP and systemic vascular resistance [36, 37]. Falkner [38] has proposed that essential hypertension in blacks is predominantly the result of increased cardiovascular reactivity and systemic vascular resistance. Also of interest is the consistent inverse association between hypertensive risk, socioeconomic status, and psychosocial stress, which has been documented by James [39]. Environmental stressors could therefore predispose black children to hypertension.

Racial differences in the renin-angiotensin-aldosterone system also exist. Plasma-renin activity is lower in black adults and children and does not rise as much in response to salt deprivation [33]. In addition, blacks with high BP tend to have lower renin levels than their hypertensive white counterparts [33]. Because sodium retention plays an important role in low-renin hypertension, it is possible that blacks have inherited a tendency toward salt-sensitive high BP. Grim has proposed that individuals most capable of retaining salt were best able to survive the severe demands of slavery in the United States and thus produced future generations of salt-sensitive individuals [40]. Exposure to high dietary salt in modern society has therefore led to the increased prevalence of essential hypertension in blacks. In support of this hypothesis are studies demonstrating greater increases in BP with salt loading in blacks than in whites [33].

Plasma aldosterone levels and urinary aldosterone excretion are substantially lower in black adults and children [41]. A chronic decrease in aldosterone could enhance vascular smooth muscle and myocardial contractility leading to high BP. Aldosterone secretion is primarily controlled by the renin-angiotensin system and potassium. The lower plasma-renin activity of blacks therefore explains, at least in part, their lower aldosterone levels. In addition, both dietary intake and urinary excretion of potassium are lower in blacks, which also contributes to relative hypoaldosteronism [40, 41]. Reduced potassium intake may be associated with high BP, and high potassium intake (3–4 g/day) has been shown to lower BP [42]. Increased potassium intake could therefore provide an important non-pharmacologic treatment for hypertensive blacks.

In addition to their higher incidence of hypertension, blacks are also at greater risk for hypertension-associated stroke, heart disease, and kidney failure. As treatment for high BP has improved, death rates for stroke and cardiovascular disease have declined. In contrast, the prevalence of renal failure due to hypertension continues to rise in blacks. Between the ages of 25 and 44 years, blacks have nearly 20 times the rate of kidney failure from high BP as whites [43].

The reasons that blacks are more vulnerable to renal injury from high BP are unclear. Genetic differences may be involved. In a retrospective study, a significant loss of renal function was found in 15% of adults with well-treated essential hypertension [44]. There were no significant differences between patients who lost renal function and those who did not, in terms of the duration of hypertension, BP levels during treatment, medication regimens, or follow-up. However, there was a significant association between loss of kidney function and race, with renal impairment occurring more than two times as frequently in blacks than in whites. This information indicates that at comparable levels of BP, blacks have a greater susceptibility to kidney damage than whites. In comparison with whites, blacks have alterations in kidney function including blunted sodium excretion, lower renal blood flow and higher renal vascular resistance, and reduced urinary kallikrein excretion [45]. These or other characteristics could cause or sustain hypertension and promote progressive renal disease. Clearly more information is needed not only about the factors that make blacks more susceptible to high BP but also about the factors that make the kidneys of black patients more susceptible to hypertensive damage.

Treatment of essential hypertension also differs in blacks and whites. Hypertensive black patients are more likely to respond to diuretics and less likely to respond to beta blockers and angiotensin-converting enzyme (ACE) inhibitors [33, 42]. The reasons for these racial differences in drug efficacy are unclear but may relate to lower levels of plasma-renin activity in blacks. Other antihypertensive drugs appear to be equally effective in blacks and whites [29]. Given the high rate of kidney failure in hypertensive blacks, it is important to recognize that the antihypertensive medication itself, and not just the reduction of BP, may have a beneficial effect on the course of progressive renal disease. Brazy and Fitzwilliam [46] have shown that specific antihypertensive medications preserve kidney function in patients with chronic renal disease better than other commonly used drugs. Further information about the use of specific antihypertensive medications to prevent progressive renal disease in hypertension is needed before definitive recommendations can be made.

Hypertension and Diabetes Mellitus

Hypertension is very common in adults with diabetes mellitus. It contributes substantially to death and disability in patients with this disease by exacerbating coronary artery disease, stoke, peripheral vascular disease, and renal failure. Physicians who care for children with diabetes mellitus rarely see these devastating long-term complications. However, current research indicates that pediatricians can influence the development of organ damage and hypertension in children with diabetes mellitus.

Hypertension is closely linked to the development of renal disease in diabetes. Therefore, an understanding of the natural history of diabetic kidney disease is important in identifying patients at risk for serious diabetic complications and for developing preventive strategies. Renal involvement in diabetes mellitus evolves through five stages [47]. Stage I is the hyperfunction-hypertrophy stage present in most patients at the time of diagnosis. Increased glomerular and kidney size are common findings. Microalbuminuria (urinary albumin excretion 30–250 mg/day) and abnormally high glomerular filtration rate (>150 ml/min/1.73 m^2) are also characteristic of this stage. These rates return toward normal with the institution of insulin therapy and can often be completely normalized with strict glycemic control. BP is normal during this stage.

Stage II, the "silent" stage, begins after about 1–3 years of diabetes duration. There is no clinical or laboratory evidence of kidney dysfunction. Histologically, glomerular enlargement, thickening of the glomerular basement membrane, and a relative expansion of the glomerular mesangium are found. BP is again usually normal. Most patients with diabetes mellitus do not progress beyond this stage even after many years of disease.

Stage III is incipient diabetic nephropathy, which typically develops after 10–15 years of diabetes. Microalbuminuria reappears and progressively increases. Glomerular filtration rate can be high or normal but gradually declines as urinary albumin excretion rises. Increased plasma prorenin concentrations may also provide a marker for evolution to this stage [48]. Elevations in BP are also first noted during this stage. Frank hypertension may or may not develop. Kidney pathology demonstrates increasing degrees of diffuse mesangial expansion. Overt diabetic nephropathy (stage IV) eventually develops in 30–40% of insulin-dependent diabetics after about 15–20 years of disease duration. Dipstick positive proteinuria (urinary albumin excretion > 250 mg/day) appears along with progressive renal insufficiency. Hypertension is usually present. Mesangial sclerosis becomes more severe with occlusion of glomerular capillaries. Eventual progression to end stage kidney disease (stage V) is inevitable at this point.

The factors involved in the transition from stage II to stage III diabetic nephropathy are unclear. Poor glycemic control appears to be a risk factor [49]. However, glycemic control alone does not accurately distinguish patients who will develop nephropathy from those who will not [50]. Because improved glycemic control slows the rate of progression of diabetic kidney disease, more intensive treatment should be offered to children with incipient nephropathy [51].

Genetic factors may also determine the risk of nephropathy. Seaquist and colleagues [52] examined diabetic siblings for clinical evidence of nephropathy. If one sibling had kidney disease, the risk of nephropathy in other siblings was 80% or more. The incidence of nephropathy was 17% in siblings of patients without renal involvement. In addition, nondiabetic parents of patients with diabetic nephropathy have higher BPs than parents of diabetic patients without renal disease, indicating that an inherited disposition to essential hypertension may be related to susceptibility to diabetic nephropathy [53]. In support of this hypothesis, increased sodium-lithium contertransport in red blood cells, a marker for essential hypertension, has been found in diabetic patients with nephropathy [54]. However, one large study failed to confirm the increased incidence of parental hypertension or red cell sodium-lithium transport in patients with diabetic nephropathy [55].

Although hypertension may not initiate diabetic nephropathy, it is clearly an important factor in its progression. Longitudinal studies have demonstrated a rise in BP of about 5% per year during the course of incipient and overt diabetic nephropathy [56]. Effective antihypertensive therapy dramatically reduces the rate of decline in glomerular filtration rate in patients with overt nephropathy and protects them from other end-organ damage [56]. The role of antihypertensive treatment for diabetic patients with incipient nephropathy and rising or borderline elevations in BP is less clear, but short-term studies suggest that such therapy can reduce microalbuminuria and potentially prevent the development of overt nephropathy

[50, 57]. Health care providers who care for children with diabetes should carefully track BP at each visit and assess urinary albumin excretion yearly after 5 years of disease duration. If pathologic albuminuria is found, serum creatinine concentration and glomerular filtration rate should be measured. Rising BP, persistent microalbuminuria, declining glomerular filtration rate, or any combination thereof is currently the best indicator available for end stage renal disease risk. Such indicators identify a subset of patients who benefit the most from aggressive glycemic control and antihypertensive treatment [50].

The etiology of nephropathy-associated hypertension in insulin-dependent diabetes is unclear [58]. Diabetics tend to have increased total body sodium and extracellular fluid volume, suggesting a salt-sensitive form of high BP. Enhanced vascular sensitivity to pressor substances (angiotensin II and norepinephrine) may also contribute. The efficacy of ACE inhibitors strongly implicates the renin-angiotensin system as a cause of high BP in diabetics. Consistent abnormalities in circulating renin activity or angiotensin II have not been demonstrated in hypertensive diabetics, although some investigators feel that these hormones are inappropriately elevated for the degree of volume expansion in these patients. Interestingly, increased plasma levels of prorenin (the precursor of active renin) are highly correlated with the subsequent development of nephropathy and other end-organ complications in children with diabetes [48].

The evaluation of children with diabetes and hypertension should proceed as described in Chapter 4. Although the coincidence of high BP and incipient or overt nephropathy are usually consistent with a diagnosis of nephropathy-associated hypertension, clinicians should remain alert for other secondary causes of hypertension in these patients. A trial of non-drug therapy is appropriate in this setting. Weight reduction (if appropriate), moderate dietary sodium restriction, and a regular aerobic exercise program may not only help lower BP but also promote better glycemic control and enhance the efficacy of antihypertensive medications [59]. The American Diabetes Association recommends that hypertensive patients with diabetes mellitus receive pharmacologic treatment if BP is severely elevated or if a trial of non-drug therapy is not effective. The goal of therapy is a BP less than 130/85 in adults and less than the ninetieth percentile for age in children [60]. ACE inhibitors are the preferred treatment for diabetic patients [60, 61]. This class of medications effectively reduces BP in most diabetics without altering glucose or lipid metabolism. In addition, these agents can reduce albuminuria and loss of renal function. The only serious side effect of these medications in diabetic patients is the potential for hyperkalemia. This complication generally arises only in patients with advanced nephropathy and renal insufficiency who have an underlying defect in urinary potassium excretion caused by hyporeninemic hypoaldosteronism.

Exercise and Hypertension

Consistent low-intensity exercise appears to reduce the risk of premature death and cardiovascular disease and may help lower BP. There is certainly no reason not to permit and encourage modest levels of physical activity in otherwise healthy patients with high BP [62]. Controversy arises when hypertensive children wish to participate in strenuous physical activity or competitive sports. Unfortunately, specific recommendations about athletic activities and hypertensive children are unavailable because no carefully controlled long-term studies of the effect of exercise on BP have been performed. Nevertheless, an understanding of currently available information can permit a reasonable approach to this issue.

BP responds differently to the two basic types of physical activity [63]. During vigorous dynamic or isotonic exercise (e.g., swimming, running, cycling), systolic BP rises dramatically while diastolic BP rises slightly or even falls (see Figure 7.1). These normal changes reflect an increase in cardiac output and a decrease in peripheral vascular resistance. During static or isometric exercise (e.g., weightlifting, gymnastics), both systolic and diastolic BPs rise, often to a higher level than during dynamic effort, reflecting an increase in both cardiac output and peripheral vascular resistance. In a study of normotensive adult body builders [64], direct intra-arterial pressure was recorded in a nonexercised limb during heavy exercise. The highest pressure was 450/310 mm Hg during a double leg press. The lowest pressure was 290/230 mm Hg during a single arm curl. Mean arterial pressure averaged 131 mm Hg during a 90-minute workout. The body appears to adapt quite well to these massive changes in BP, which in different circumstances would be associated with a hypertensive crisis.

Hypertensive patients experience similar changes in BP during exercise and, therefore, generally have higher peak pressures than their normotensive counterparts (Figure 7.2). Concern that these extreme pressure levels might be harmful led a panel of experts sponsored by the American College of Cardiology and the National Heart, Lung, and Blood Institute to formulate specific guidelines regarding participation of hypertensive patients in competitive sports [65]. Their recommendations are summarized in Table 7.1.

Restriction from athletic activities should ideally be based on evidence that abrupt elevations in BP place the hypertensive individual at higher risk for a catastrophic event, exacerbate hypertensive organ damage, or contribute to sustained high BP. Retrospective studies of individuals who died during athletic activities suggest that patients with hypertension are at higher risk for exercise-related sudden death [62, 63]. These individuals are typically middle-aged and have underlying coronary artery disease. Hypertension has never been implicated in the exercise-related death of a young athlete, and there is no convincing evidence that exercise-induced pressure elevations are harmful in the absence of ischemic heart disease

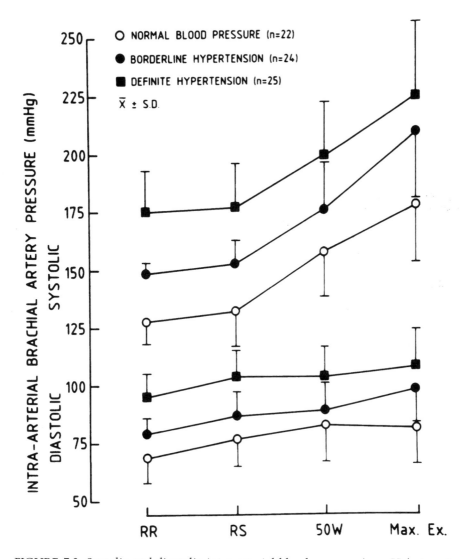

FIGURE 7.2. Systolic and diastolic intra-arterial blood pressure (mm Hg) at supine rest (RR), sitting rest (RS), 50-watt exercise (50W), and maximal exercise (Max. Ex.) in subjects with normal blood pressure, borderline hypertension, and definite hypertension. (Reproduced with permission from R Fagard, E Bielen, P Hespel, et al. Physical Exercise and Hypertension. In JH Laragh, BM Brenner [eds], Hypertension: Pathophysiology, Diagnosis and Management. New York: Raven, 1990;1985.)

[65, 66]. Nevertheless, it seems prudent to avoid strenuous dynamic or static exercise and to restrict competitive sports participation to low-intensity activities in severely hypertensive children until their BPs are controlled. This recommendation is consistent with that of the 1987 Task Force

TABLE 7.1
Recommendations for Participation in Competitive Sports[a] for the Pediatric Hypertensive Patient [42, 65]

---

1. Children with significant hypertension and no evidence of target-organ involvement[b] can participate in all competitive sports. These children should have their blood pressure remeasured at least every 2 months to monitor the impact of competition.
2. Children with severe hypertension who do not have target-organ involvement should be restricted, particularly from high static sports[c], until their high blood pressure is controlled.
3. The eligibility for participation in competitive athletics for children with hypertension and target-organ damage or other cardiovascular diseases should be determined on an individual basis based on severity of both their hypertension and associated conditions.

---

[a]A *competitive athlete* is one who participates in an organized team or individual sport that requires competition against others as a central component, places a high premium on excellence and achievement, and requires vigorous training in a systematic fashion.
[b]Criteria for target-organ disease include the following: (1) Cardiac involvement is present if there is (a) clinical, electrocardiographic, or radiologic evidence of coronary artery disease; (b) left ventricular hypertrophy or "strain" by electrocardiography or left ventricular hypertrophy by echocardiography; or (c) left ventricular dysfunction or cardiac failure. (2) Renal involvement is present if there is pathologic proteinuria or the glomerular filtration rate is less than normal. (3) Eye involvement is present if retinal hemorrhages or exudates are seen. (4) Cerebrovascular involvement is present if there is a history of transient ischemic attacks or stroke. (5) Peripheral vascular involvement is present if there is absence of one or more major pulses in the extremities with or without claudication or an aneurysm.
[c]High static sports include field events (throwing), gymnastics, karate/judo, water skiing, weight lifting, body building, downhill skiing, wrestling, boxing, cycling, decathlon, rowing, and speed skating.

Report on Blood Pressure Control in Children [1]. The American Academy of Pediatrics has recently proposed that hypertensive children avoid weight and power lifting, body building, and strength training [67].

Although the risks of exercise in hypertensive patients remain unclear, there is reasonable evidence from adequately controlled studies that dynamic exercise can lower BP in hypertensive adults. In reviews of available research [62, 63], sustained endurance training has been found to reduce resting BP by approximately 10 mm Hg in both systolic and diastolic levels. Similar improvements in BP control have also been documented in hypertensive adolescents [68]. In the absence of uncontrolled severe hypertension or other diseases that would make strenuous activity unwise, medically supervised dynamic exercise or competitive sports can be recommended as a potentially effective nonpharmacologic therapy for high BP in children [65, 69]. It should be noted that physical training programs leading to BP reduction generally require 30 minutes or more of relatively intense exercise performed at least three times per week, and that the beneficial effect of such training gradually dissipates when discontinued.

The long-term effect of intensive strength training or static exercise on BP is undetermined. Although it has been stated that weight-lifting tends to produce high BP, there is no evidence that the acute severe elevations in BP caused by static exercise causes or exacerbates chronic hypertension [62, 70]. Most studies in adults suggest that weight training does not alter resting BP [62, 63]. Limited information indicates that children respond in a similar fashion [70]. It may, therefore, be unreasonable to block the promising career of a hypertensive weight lifter, shot putter, or wrestler. In this situation, the best approach may be to recommend dynamic and static exercise, especially circuit weight training. Hagberg and colleagues [71] have shown that weight training in hypertensive adolescents appears to maintain BP reductions achieved by running and can decrease BP even further.

Before exercise is recommended or vigorous athletic competition is permitted, hypertensive children should be evaluated as described in Chapter 4. This evaluation must include an assessment for cardiovascular abnormalities associated with sports-related sudden death, such as hypertrophic cardiomyopathy, congenital or acquired cases of coronary artery disease, aortic stenosis, mitral valve prolapse, carditis, arrythmias, and Marfan's syndrome [72, 73]. Careful questioning about exercise-associated syncope, light-headedness, or chest pain, and a family history of syncope or sudden death, hypertrophic cardiomyopathy, or premature atherosclerotic heart disease may provide the only clue that a potentially lethal disorder exists. Electrocardiograms or echocardiograms are probably not necessary unless indicated for other reasons. If these tests are obtained, their interpretation must take into account the normal physiologic changes in cardiac structure and function that occur in well-conditioned athletes [74]. Failure to recognize these changes can lead to unnecessary additional evaluation or unwarranted proscription of athletic activities.

The role of exercise stress testing in the evaluation of hypertensive children for sports participation is unclear. There is no solid evidence that high BP in itself makes exercise dangerous, or that specific peak levels of BP during exercise are unhealthy. In addition, it is difficult to simulate the cardiovascular demands of various athletic activities using standardized stress test protocols. Children exercise at various levels of intensity and different sports impose different hemodynamic stresses on the cardiovascular system [75]. Although the 1987 Task Force downplays the value of stress testing in hypertensive patients, several experts suggest that it be performed before sanctioning athletic activities [1, 75, 76]. We currently recommend stress testing for all patients with sustained mild to moderate hypertension before allowing participation in strenuous sports, and for all patients with severe hypertension after BP has been controlled before endorsing any type of exercise program. These patients should probably be restudied periodically to exclude evolving cardiac dysfunction. The development of serious arrythmias, ischemia, or hypotension during exercise testing indicates that strenuous sports should be avoided. The significance of marked BP increases during testing is unclear with regard to eligibility for athletic competition [65]. We realize that these recommendations are controversial and may not be widely accepted. Nevertheless, we believe that exercise stress testing is valuable for counseling and reassuring hypertensive children and their families that participation in strenuous physical activity and competitive athletics is safe.

A final consideration in the management of the hypertensive athlete is selection of appropriate medications for those who require pharmacologic treatment. Some patients may experience problems with various antihypertensive drugs. For example, short-term treatment with diuretics can impair maximal oxygen uptake during exercise and worsen the performance in distance runners. Depletion of intravascular volume appears to be responsible for these adverse effects [63]. There are no data on the effects of chronic diuretic treatment on exercise capacity; however, depletion of potassium or other electrolytes could potentially alter muscle function. Beta-adrenergic blocking agents, especially nonselective ones, appear to markedly reduce capacity for prolonged submaximal exercise and may therefore be inappropriate for children engaged in endurance training or dynamic sports [63]. Physicians who care for these children are urged to watch for medication-induced deterioration in physical performance. A variety of drugs with different mechanisms of action are available for treating high BP. In most cases, it is possible to control BP and preserve exercise tolerance through careful medication selection and patient follow-up. Angiotensin-converting enzyme inhibitors and calcium channel blockers seem to be the most effective in lowering BP without impairing hemodynamic response to vigorous exercise [63].

References

1. Report of the Second Task Force on Blood Pressure Control in Children. Pediatrics 1987;79:1.
2. Messerli FH. Obesity in hypertension: how innocent a bystander? Am J Med 1984;77:1077.
3. Feld LG, Springate JE. Hypertension in children. Curr Probl Pediatr 1988;18:319.
4. Gortmaker SL, Dietz WH, Sobol AM, Wehler CA. Increasing pediatric obesity in the United States. Am J Dis Child 1987;141:535.
5. Dornfeld LP, Maxwell MH, Waks A, Tuck M. Mechanisms of hypertension in obesity. Kidney Int 1987;32:254.
6. Dustan HP. Obesity and hypertension. Diabetes Care 1991;14:488.
7. Rocchini AP, Katch V, Anderson J, et al. Blood pressure in obese adolescents: effect of weight loss. Pediatrics 1988;82:16.
8. Rocchini AP, Key J, Bondie D, et al. The effect of weight loss on the sensitivity of blood pressure to sodium in obese adolescents. N Engl J Med 1989;321:580.

9. Landsberg L. Insulin and hypertension: lessons from obesity. N Engl J Med 1987;317:378.
10. DeFronzo RA, Ferrannini E. Insulin resistance: a multi-faceted syndrome responsible for NIDDM, obesity, hypertension, dyslipidemia and atherosclerotic cardiovascular disease. Diabetes Care 1991;14:173.
11. Maxwell MH, Schroth PC, Waks AU, et al. Error in blood-pressure measurement due to incorrect cuff size in obese patients. Lancet 1982;2:33.
12. Lohman TG. Research progress in validation of laboratory methods of assessing body composition. Med Sci Sports Exerc 1984;16:596.
13. Hammer LD, Kraemer HC, Wilson DM, et al. Standardized percentile curves of body-mass index for children and adolescents. Am J Dis Child 1991;145:259.
14. National Institutes of Health Consensus Development Conference. Statement on the health implications of obesity. Ann Intern Med 1985;103:1073.
15. Dietz WH. Prevention of childhood obesity. Pediatr Clin North Am 1986;33:823.
16. Ross RD, Daniels SR, Loggie JMH, et al. Sleep apnea-associated hypertension and reversible left ventricular hypertrophy. J Pediatr 1987;111:253.
17. Hoffstein V, Chan CK, Slutsky AS. Sleep apnea and systemic hypertension: a causal association review. Am J Med 1991;91:190.
18. Lake CR, Gallant S, Masson E, Miller P. Adverse drug effects attributed to phenylpropanolamine: a review of 142 case reports. Am J Med 1990;89:195.
19. Bravo EL. Phenylpropanolamine. In JH Laragh, BM Brenner (eds), Hypertension: Pathophysiology, Diagnosis and Management. New York: Raven, 1990;1911.
20. Lake CR, Zaloga G, Bray J, et al. Transient hypertension after two phenylpropanolamine diet aids and the effects of caffeine: a placebo controlled follow-up study. Am J Med 1989;86:427.
21. Bradley JG. Nonprescription drugs and hypertension: which ones affect blood pressure. Postgrad Med 1991;89:195.
22. Coates ML, Rembold CM, Farr BM. Does pseudoephedrine increase blood pressure in patients with controlled hypertension? J Fam Pract 1995;40:22.
23. Gadomski A, Horton L. The need for rational therapeutics in the use of cough and cold medicine in infants. Pediatrics 1992;89:774.
24. Shearin RB, Boehlke JR. Hormonal contraception. Pediatr Clin North Am 1989;36:697.
25. Baird DT, Glasier AF. Hormonal contraception. N Engl J Med 1993;328:1543.
26. MacFarlane LL, Orak DJ, Simpson WM. NSAIDs, antihypertensive agents and loss of blood pressure control. Am Fam Physician 1995;51:849.
27. Mortensen ME, Rennebohm RM. Clinical pharmacology and use of nonsteroidal anti-inflammatory drugs. Pediatr Clin North Am 1989;36:1113.
28. Oates JA, Fitzgerald GA, Branch RA, et al. Clinical implications of prostaglandin and thromboxane A_2 formation. N Engl J Med 1988;319:761.
29. Oates JA. Cyclo-Oxygenase Inhibitors and Blood Pressure. In JH Laragh, BM Brenner (eds), Hypertension: Pathophysiology, Diagnosis and Management. New York: Raven, 1990;1905.

30. Patrono C, Dunn MJ. The clinical significance of inhibition of renal prostaglandin synthesis. Kidney Int 1987;32:1.
31. Radack KL, Deck CC, Bloomfield SS. Ibuprofen interferes with the efficacy of antihypertensive drugs. Ann Intern Med 1987;107:628.
32. Wong DG, Lamki L, Spence JD, et al. Effect of non-steroidal anti-inflammatory drugs on control of hypertension by beta-blockers and diuretics. Lancet 1986;1:997.
33. Savage DD, Watkins LO, Grim CE, Kumanyika SK. Hypertension in Black Populations. In JH Laragh, BM Brenner (eds), Hypertension: Pathophysiology, Diagnosis and Management. New York: Raven, 1990;1837.
34. Hediger ML, Schall JI, Katz SH, et al. Resting blood pressure and pulse rate distributions in black adolescents. Pediatrics 1984;74:1016.
35. Kozinetz CA. Sexual maturation and blood pressure levels of a biracial sample of girls. Am J Dis Child 1991;145:142.
36. Arensman FW, Treiber FA, Gruber MP, Strong WB. Exercise-incuded differences in cardiac output, blood pressure and systemic vascular resistance in a healthy biracial population of 10 year old boys. Am J Dis Child 1989;143:212.
37. Treiber FA, Musante L, Strong WB, Levy M. Racial differences in young children's blood pressure. Am J Dis Child 1989;143:720.
38. Falkner B. Is there black hypertension? Hypertension 1987;10:551.
39. James SA. Psychosocial and Environmental Factors in Black Hypertension. In WD Hall, E Saunders, N Shulman (eds), Hypertension in Blacks. Chicago: Year Book, 1985;132.
40. Grim CE, Luft FC, Miller JZ. Racial differences in blood pressure in Evans County, Georgia: relationship to sodium and potassium intake and plasma renin activity. J Chronic Dis 1980;33:87.
41. Pratt JH, Jones JJ, Miller JZ, et al. Racial differences in aldosterone excretion and plasma aldosterone concentrations in children. N Engl J Med 1989;321:1152.
42. The Fifth Report of the Joint National Committee on Detection, Evaluation, and Treatment of High Blood Pressure. Arch Intern Med 1993;153:154.
43. Gordon D. Racial differences in ESRD. Dialysis and Transplantation 1990; 19:114.
44. Rostand SG, Brown G, Kirk KA, et al. Renal insufficiency in treated essential hypertension. N Engl J Med 1989;320:684.
45. Dustan HP, Curtis JJ, Luke RG, Rostand SG. Systemic hypertension and the kidney in black patients. Am J Cardiol 1987;60:731.
46. Brazy PC, Fitzwilliam JF. Progressive renal disease: role of race and antihypertensive medications. Kidney Int 1990;37:1113.
47. Mogensen CE. Prediction of clinical diabetic nephropathy in insulin-dependent diabetes mellitus patients. Diabetes 1990;39:761.
48. Daneman D, Crompton CH, Balfe JW, et al. Plasma prorenin as an early marker of nephropathy in diabetic adolescents. Kidney Int 1994;46:1154.
49. Bojestig M, Arnqvist HJ, Hermasson G, et al. Declining incidence of nephropathy in insulin-dependent diabetes mellitus. N Engl J Med 1994;330:15.

50. Lane P, Steffes M, Mauer SM. The role of the pediatric nephrologist in the care of children with diabetes mellitus. Pediatr Nephrol 1991;5:359.
51. Krolewski AS, Lori MB, Krolewski M, et al. Glycosylated hemoglobin and the risk of microalbuminuria in patients with insulin-dependent diabetes mellitus. N Engl J Med 1995;332:1251.
52. Seaquist ER, Goetz FC, Rich S, Barbosa J. Familial clustering of diabetic kidney disease. N Engl J Med 1989;320:1161.
53. Krolewski AS, Canessa M, Warram JH, et al. Predisposition to hypertension and susceptibility to renal disease in insulin-dependent diabetes mellitus. N Engl J Med 1988;318:140.
54. Mangili R, Bending JJ, Scott G, et al. Increased sodium-lithium countertransport activity in red cells of patients with insulin-dependent diabetes and nephropathy. N Engl J Med 1988;318:146.
55. Jensen JS, Mathiesen ER, Norgaard K, et al. Increased blood pressure and erythrocyte sodium/lithium countertransport activity are not inherited in diabetic nephropathy. Diabetologia 1990;33:619.
56. Mogensen CE. Management of the Diabetic Patient with Hypertension. In JH Laragh, BM Brenner (eds), Hypertension: Pathophysiology, Diagnosis and Management. New York: Raven, 1990;1717.
57. Cook J, Daneman D, Spino M, et al. Angiotensin converting enzyme inhibitor therapy to decrease microalbuminuria in normotensive children with insulin-dependent diabetes mellitus. J Pediatr 1990;117:39.
58. Stern N, Tuck ML. Mechanisms of Hypertension in Diabetes Mellitus. In JH Laragh, BM Brenner (eds), Hypertension: Pathophysiology, Diagnosis and Management. New York: Raven, 1990;1689.
59. Tjoa HI, Kaplan NM. Nonpharmacological treatment of hypertension in diabetes mellitus. Diabetes Care 1991;14:449.
60. American Diabetes Association. Standards of medical care for patients with diabetes mellitus. Diabetes Care 1995;18(Suppl 1):8.
61. Lewis EJ, Hunsicker LG, Bain RP, Rohde RD. The effect of angiotensin converting enzyme inhibition on diabetic nephropathy. N Engl J Med 1993;329:1456.
62. American College of Sports Medicine. Physical activity, physical fitness and hypertension. Med Sci Sports Exerc 1993;25:i.
63. Fagard R, Bielen E, Hespel P, et al. Physical Exercise and Hypertension. In JH Laragh, BM Brenner (eds), Hypertension: Pathophysiology, Diagnosis and Management. New York: Raven, 1990;1985.
64. MacDougall D. Direct measurement of arterial blood pressure during heavy resistance training. Med Sci Sports Exerc 1983;15:158.
65. Maron BJ, Mitchell JH. 26th Bethesda Conference: recommendations for determining eligibility for competition in athletes with cardiovascular abnormalities. J Am Coll Cardiol 1994;24:846.
66. Maron BJ, Roberts WC, McAllister HA, et al. Sudden death in young athletes. Circulation 1980;62:218.

67. American Academy of Pediatrics Committee on Sports Medicine and Fitness. Medical conditions affecting sports participation. Pediatrics 1994;94:757.
68. Hagberg JM, Goldring D, Ehsani AA, et al. Effect of exercise training on blood pressure and hemodynamic features of hypertensive adolescents. Am J Cardiol 1983;52:763.
69. Somers VK, Conway J, Johnston J. Effects of endurance training on baroreflex sensitivity and blood pressure in borderline hypertension. Lancet 1991; 1:1363.
70. Webb DR. Strength training in children and adolescents. Pediatr Clin North Am 1990;37:1187.
71. Hagberg JM, Ehsoni AA, Goldring D. Effect of weight training on blood pressure and hemodynamics in hypertensive adolescents. J Pediatr 1984;104:147.
72. Driscoll DJ. Cardiovascular evaluation of the child and adolescent before participation in sports. Mayo Clin Proc 1985;60:867.
73. Neuspiel DR. Sudden death from myocardititis in young athletes. Mayo Clin Proc 1986;61:226.
74. Huston TP, Puffer JC, Rodney WM. The athletic heart syndrome. N Engl J Med 1985;313:24.
75. Freed MD. Recreational and sports recommendations for the child with heart disease. Pediatr Clin North Am 1984;31:1307.
76. Portman RJ, Robson AM. Controversies in Pediatric Hypertension. In BM Tune, SA Mendoza (eds), Contemporary Issues in Nephrology. Vol 12. New York: Churchill Livingstone, 1984;265.

CHAPTER 8

Common Questions About Blood Pressure in Childhood

Leonard G. Feld

Questions and Cases for the Practitioner

The following is a series of answers to the most common questions (referrals) concerning hypertension in childhood. The questions and referrals were obtained from primary care practitioners in the Western New York region.

1. *When should blood pressure (BP) measurements be made in children?* The Report of the Task Force on Blood Pressure Control in Children recommends yearly BP determinations from 3 years of age. The authors of this book agree with this recommendation. This standard is for healthy children. Any ill-appearing infants or children should have a BP measurement. As discussed in Chapter 2, there are a number of methods to determine BP in infants and small children. There are seven cuff sizes for ausculatory and oscillometric instruments (see Table 2.1, Chapter 2).

2. *Are orthostatic BPs useful or accurate in pediatric patients?* Yes. It is possible to reliably measure orthostatic BPs from about 6 months of age. *Orthostatic hypotension* is defined as a greater than 10 mm Hg fall in BP. It usually implies a significant (>20%) reduction in circulating blood volume. The method for determining if orthostatic hypotension has occured is as follows: (1) determine the first BP in the recumbant position; (2) determine the second reading in the sitting position after a stabilization period of at least 2 minutes; and

(3) determine the third reading in the standing position after a stabilization period of at least 2 minutes.

3. *If a patient has an elevated BP, how frequently should the patient be seen in the office?* It depends on whether the level of BP is above the ninetieth, ninety-fifth, or ninety-ninth percentile for age.

    a. If the BP is between the ninetieth and ninety-fifth percentile and the child is asymptomatic, repeat readings should be performed once a month for 3 months. If the child is overweight, this provides an opportunity to initiate a weight control and exercise program.

    b. If the BP is greater than the ninety-fifth percentile but less than the ninety-ninth percentile and the child is asymptomatic, repeat readings should be performed once a week for 2 weeks. **After that time phase I should be started if the child is not overweight (see Figure 4.1, Chapter 4).** If the child is overweight, this provides an opportunity to initiate a weight control and exercise program. *Points of caution*—do *not* limit the history or physical examination because the child is overweight; and do *not* attribute obesity to the inability to appreciate femoral or distal pulses—coarctation occurs in obese children.

    c. If the BP is greater than the ninety-ninth percentile for age, an immediate evaluation is required. The child may require admission to the hospital for frequent monitoring and possible therapy.

4. *When should a hypertensive child be referred to a pediatric nephrologist, pediatric endocrinologist, or pediatric cardiologist?* The answer is largely dependent on the comfort level of the practitioner. If the phase approach is used, the referral can be deferred until phase 2 or 3. In cases of severe or symptomatic hypertension (>ninety-ninth percentile for age), immediate consultation is recommended. Depending on the region of the country, the majority of the hypertensive patient referrals may be directed to either a pediatric nephrologist, pediatric endocrinologist, or pediatric cardiologist. Regardless of the referral pattern, subspecialists are available to assist for the evaluation and to prevent unnecessary testing.

5. *When should the patient start medications?* If the patient has a BP greater than the ninety-fifth percentile for age and sex and is not obese, pharmacologic therapy is recommended. If the child is obese, a nonpharmacologic approach is indicated unless the child is symptomatic. If the decision is not to treat, the child requires frequent monitoring in the office, school, or home. The family should understand the benefits, risks, side effects, contraindications, and alternatives to treatment. It is mandatory to provide a complete description of the major side effects. **Make the patient and family part of the decision and treatment process.** If the patient and family monitors the BP at home and in school, they need written instructions with BP limits,

which indicate when to call the physician and when to hold the medication for low BPs. For example:

Call the Kidney Center if your BP is greater than:

Systolic (upper number) > (*add ninety-fifth percentile for age and sex*) mm Hg, or

Diastolic (lower number) > (*add ninety-fifth percentile for age and sex*) mm Hg

Hold the medication and call the Kidney Center if your BP is less than:

Systolic (upper number) < 110 mm Hg (dependent on age) or

Diastolic (lower number) < 60 mm Hg (dependent on age)

6. *When is the diagnosis of hypertension made?* It is essential to use judgment before assigning any diagnosis to patients. The label "hypertensive child" may limit the child's ability to participate in sports, to obtain life or medical insurance, or to obtain employment. In some school districts, the issue of liability is overwhelming. Despite the physician's best efforts and documentation, participation in competitive sports may be precluded in a child with the diagnosis of hypertension. If the child is obese, use the diagnosis of obesity before giving the diagnosis of hypertension. By explaining the issue of school liability to the child and family, there may be improved compliance with weight reduction. If the child is hypertensive (>ninety-fifth percentile for age), is not obese, and is on medication, the chart should reflect normalization of BP with medication. Over time, this documentation assists in many aspects of school and work life. When the time comes for life insurance, 2 years or more in therapy should provide no obstacle to insurability at standard rates.

Case Studies

Case 1: The Child with Systolic Hypertension and Obesity

John is a 13-year-old boy. Hypertension was noted for the first time on a routine physical examination for high school football. He has been examined regularly by his physician since 4 years of age. He has never been sick, and only had an inguinal hernia repair at age 5. John's BP ranged from 170/65 to 175/75 mm Hg on three readings over a 1-month period. One year before his private doctor visit, the school recorded a systolic BP of 190 mm Hg before the basketball season. Because John was the team leader, this information was not communicated by the school or family to his physician. John's past medical and family history are unremarkable. His physical exam is normal except for a BP of 175/72 mm Hg.

Questions

1. What is the differential diagnosis?
2. What laboratory or x-ray studies, if any, should be performed before the consultation?
3. What are the therapeutic options for this adolescent?
4. Should he be permitted to play team sports? Who should make the decision about his participation: private physician, cardiologist, nephrologist, school physician, family, or lawyer?

Answers

1. The child has systolic hypertension. The causes of systolic hypertension include obesity, anemia, hyperthyroidism, arteriovenous malformations, anxiety, and essential hypertension. If there is no evidence for the organic causes of systolic hypertension in the young man, essential hypertension is the most likely choice.

2. The diagnostic evaluation should be limited in scope. It is reasonable to perform a phase I evaluation (see Table 4.1, Chapter 4). However, no laboratory studies in face of an unremarkable review of systems and a normal physical examination is a reasonable approach.

3. The decision to treat systolic hypertension is quite difficult. Since his systolic value is 25% above the ninety-fifth percentile for age and sex, John has moderate hypertension, and therapy with an angiotensin-converting enzyme inhibitor or a calcium channel–blocking agent is recommended.

4. John should participate in team sports. It is important not to make children, adolescents, and young adults "hypertensive cripples." As discussed in Chapter 7, the recommendations to participate in sports are as follows:

All competitive sports	Mild to moderate hypertension (therapy) and no target-organ damage
Low-intensity sports	Mild to moderate hypertension (no therapy) Mild to moderate hypertension (therapy) and target-organ damage Severe hypertension (therapy) and no target-organ damage Severe hypertension (therapy) and target-organ damage

There is no clear answer about who should decide whether John should be permitted to participate in team sports. The physicians should provide complete information to the family. The family should make the final decision. In some cases, a laboratory and radiographic evaluation assists in the decision-making process. An echocardiogram and, in selected cases, a stress (with or without thallium) test provides more assurance to the family and school.

Case 2: The Young Child with Significant Hypertension and a Strong Family History of Hypertension

Susan is a three-year-old girl with a vibratory systolic murmur grade II/VI along the left sternal border. Her BP ranges from 134/90 to 148/94. Susan's past medical history is not contributory. Her family history is significant for hypertension on the paternal side. The father, his two brothers, one sister, and mother have hypertension. The father was diagnosed with hypertension 15 years ago, of which he maintains fair control with a beta blocker. Susan's physical examination is normal except for blood pressues readings ranging from 124/72 to 128/82, without a change in the lower extremities.

Questions

1. Does the patient have hypertension and if so, how significant is it?
2. What is the differential diagnosis?
3. What laboratory or x-ray studies, if any, should be performed before the consultation?
4. What are the therapeutic options?

Answers

1. The approach is to refer to the tables for BP based on age and sex (see Tables 2.2 and 2.3, Chapter 2). The short cut is to use the "Pearls of Hypertension" (see Chapter 2).

Definition of hypertension (>ninety-fifth percentile for age and sex):

If systolic BP equals or exceeds: $[100 + (3.0 \times \text{patient age [in years]})]$

If diastolic BP equals or exceeds: $[70 + (1.5 \times \text{patient age [in years]})]$

Classification of hypertension

Mild	1–15% above ninety-fifth percentile for age and sex
Moderate	16–30% above ninety-fifth percentile for age and sex
Severe	31–50% above ninety-fifth percentile for age and sex
Emergency	50% or more above ninety-fifth percentile for age and sex

This child has hypertension, which requires a diagnostic evaluation.

2. With moderate hypertension and a strong family history of hypertension, the child requires a very detailed and planned work-up. The most likely causes of hypertension include essential hypertension, renovascular hypertension, or glucocorticoid-remediable hypertension. The diagnosis of essential hypertension is one of exclusion.

3. Renovascular hypertension should be evaluated using the algorithm (see Figure 4.2, Chapter 4). Glucocorticoid-remediable hypertension is suggested by a strong family history, relatively low plasma-renin acitivity (<0.5 ng/ml/hour), low or low-normal serum potassium concentration, and increased urinary excretion of 18-hydro-oxycortisol and 18-oxycortisol.

4. Pharmacologic therapy for glucocorticoid-remediable hypertension involves physiologic doses of hydrocortisone (7–12 mg/m^2/day) or amiloride (2.5–5.0 mg/day). Response is assessed by normalization of BP and plasma renin activity.

APPENDIX

Key Figures and Tables

See the selected chapters for additional information and references.

Definition and Measurement of Blood Pressure

Recommended Bladder Dimensions for Blood Pressure Cuff

Arm Circumference at Midpoint[a] (cm)	Cuff Name	Bladder Width (cm)	Bladder Length (cm)
5.0–7.5	Newborn	3	5
7.5–13	Infant	5	8
13–20	Child	8	13
17–26	Small adult	11	17
24–32	Adult	13	24
32–42	Large adult	17	32
42–50[b]	Thigh	20	42

[a]Midpoint of arm is defined as half the distance from the acromion to the olecranon.
[b]In large individuals (>ninety-fifth percentile for weight), the indirect blood pressure should be measured in the leg or forearm.
From Chapter 2; Table 2.1

According to a bedside pearl (Alan Gruskin Criteria) for defining hypertension in pediatrics (>ninety-fifth percentile for sex and age), the child is hypertensive if:

The systolic BP > 100 + [3.0 × patient's age in years]

The diastolic BP > 70 + [1.5 × patient's age in years]

and/or

The blood pressure > 140/90 for adolescents 14 years of age or older.

(See Chapter 2.)

A bedside pearl (Alan Gruskin Criteria) for classification of hypertension in pediatrics is:

Mild hypertension	Blood pressure is 1–15% above the ninety-fifth percentile for age and sex.
Moderate hypertension	Blood pressure is 16–30% above the ninety-fifth percentile for age and sex.
Severe hypertension	Blood pressure is 31–50% above the ninety-fifth percentile for age and sex.
Emergency	Blood pressure is greater than 50% above the ninety-fifth percentile for age and sex.

Classification of Hypertension by Age Group

Age Group	Significant Hypertension (mm Hg)	Severe Hypertension (mm Hg)
Newborn		
7 days	Systolic BP ≥96	Systolic BP ≥106
8–30 days	Systolic BP ≥104	Systolic BP ≥110
Infant (<2 yrs)	Systolic BP ≥112	Systolic BP ≥118
	Diastolic BP ≥74	Diastolic BP ≥82
Children (3–5 yrs)	Systolic BP ≥116	Systolic BP ≥124
	Diastolic BP ≥76	Diastolic BP ≥84
Children (6–9 yrs)	Systolic BP ≥122	Systolic BP ≥130
	Diastolic BP ≥78	Diastolic BP ≥86
Children (10–12 yrs)	Systolic BP ≥126	Systolic BP ≥134
	Diastolic BP ≥82	Diastolic BP ≥90
Adolescents (13–15 yrs)	Systolic BP ≥136	Systolic BP ≥144
	Diastolic BP ≥86	Diastolic BP ≥92
Adolescents (16–18 yrs)	Systolic BP ≥142	Systolic BP ≥150
	Diastolic BP ≥92	Diastolic BP ≥98

From Chapter 2, Table 2.4

Causes of Hypertension

Causes of Secondary Hypertension in the Newborn

Vascular
    Renal artery thrombosis
    Renal artery stenosis
    Renal vein thrombosis
    Aortic thrombosis
    Coarctation of the aorta
Kidney
    Acute renal failure
    Renal cortical/medullary necrosis
    Renal hypoplasia/dysplasia
    Renal tumors
    Obstructive uropathy
    Congenital nephrosis
    Autosomal recessive polycystic kidney disease
Medications
    Corticosteroids
    Ocular phenylephrine
    Narcotic-addicted mothers
    Cocaine
    Theophylline
    Pancuronium
Miscellaneous
    Fluid overload
    Increased intracranial pressure
    Pneumothorax
    Birth asphyxia
    Congenital adrenal hyperplasia
    Hyperaldosteronism
    Hypercalcemia
    Thyrotoxicosis
    Bronchopulmonary dysplasia
    Genitourinary tract surgery/omphalocele repair
    Extracorporeal membrane oxygenation
    Urinoma
    Adrenal hemorrhage
    Neuroblastoma
    Essential hypertension (rare)

From Chapter 3, Table 3.3

Secondary Causes of Hypertension in Older Infants and Children

---

Obesity
Renal disease
    Acute and chronic glomerulopathies
    Acute glomerulonephritis

(continued)

Nephrotic syndrome
Alport's syndrome
Acute renal failure
Renal cortical or medullary necrosis
Hemolytic-uremic syndrome
Henoch-Schönlein purpura
Systemic lupus erythematosus
Chronic renal failure and insufficiency
Renal hypoplasia
Obstructive uropathy
Reflux nephropathy and chronic pyelonephritis
Cystic kidney disease
Nephropathy secondary to diabetes mellitus, sickle cell disease, or interstitial nephritis
Post–renal trauma
Renal infarction
Post–renal transplant
Vascular disease
Coarctation of the aorta
Hypoplastic aorta
Marfan's syndrome
Crossed renal ectopia
Subacute bacterial endocarditis
Aortic valve insufficiency
Fibromuscular dysplasia
Neurofibromatosis
William's syndrome
Atherosclerosis (progeria, inborn error of lipid metabolism)
Takayasu's arteritis/arteritis
Renal artery stenosis/aneurysm/fistula
Renal artery compression (secondary to tumor or hematoma)
Aortic thrombosis
Renal vein thrombosis
Arteriovenous fistula
Renal transplantation (rejection, drugs)
Endocrine
Cushing's syndrome
Idiopathic primary hyperaldosteronism
Glucocorticoid remediable (dexamethasone-suppressible) hypertension
Mineralocorticoid excess (congenital adrenal hyperplasia, 17α-hydroxylase and
    11β-hydroxylase deficiencies, licorice ingestion)
Hyperthyroidism
Liddle's syndrome
Hyperparathyroidism, hypercalcemia, vitamin D intoxication
Gordon's syndrome
Tumor
Wilms' tumor
Tuberous sclerosis
Hemangiopericytoma (renin-secreting)

Pheochromocytoma (isolated or associated with multiple endocrinopathy syndrome, neurofibromatosis, or von Hippel-Lindau disease)
  Neuroblastoma and related neurogenic tumors
  Ovarian tumor
  Conn's syndrome
Drugs and toxins (see Chapter 4)
  Oral contraceptive pills
  Corticosteroids and adrenocorticotropic hormone
  Sympathomimetics (nose or eye drops, "cold" or "flu" medications)
  Amphetamines
  Methylphenidate
  Imipramine
  Clonidine withdrawal
  Metoclopramide
  Cyclosporine
  Methotrexate
  Theophylline
  Nonsteroidal anti-inflammatory agents
  Cisplatin
  Recombinant human erythropoietin
  Recreational drugs
  Lead
  Mercury
  Scorpion envenomation
  Cigarette smoking
  Caffeine
Neurologic
  Increased intracranial pressure
  Head injury or stroke
  Guillain-Barré syndrome
  Autonomic dysreflexia (spinal cord damage)
  Posterior fossa lesions
  Neurofibromatosis
  Poliomyelitis
  Dysautonomia
Other
  Sleep apnea
  Traction-induced immobilization
  Severe burns
  Genitourinary tract surgery
  Anemia (systolic)
  Asphyxia
  Pneumothorax
  Ventilator therapy
  Pregnancy
  Intravascular volume overload
  Pain, anxiety, or stress
  Alpha$_1$-antitrypsin deficiency from liver transplantation
  Asphyxiating thoracic dystrophy (Jeune syndrome)

From Chapter 3, Table 3.4

Causes of Hypertension by Underlying Factor

Coarctation of the aorta
Renin-dependent hypertension
   Renal vascular disease
   Renal parenchymal disease
   Renal tumor
   Hyperthyroidism
   Genitourinary surgery
   Unilateral hydronephrosis
   Mercury
   Oral contraceptive pills
Hypervolemia
   Acute renal failure
   Chronic renal failure
   Excess blood, plasma, or saline
   Bilateral ureteropelvic junction obstruction
   Lead
   Nonsteroidal anti-inflammatory agents
   Corticosteroids
Acute hypovolemia
   Nephrotic syndrome relapse
   Burns
   Renal, adrenal, and gastrointestinal salt loss
Catecholamine excess
   Pheochromocytoma
   Neuroblastoma
   Hypercalcemia
   Lead
   Cigarettes
   Traction-induced immobilization
   Increased sympathetic nervous system
      Guillain-Barré syndrome
      Poliomyelitis
      Dysautomia
Corticosteroid excess
   Congenital adrenal hyperplasia
   Conn's syndrome
   Cushing's syndrome
   Low-renin hypertensive states
   Cigarettes
Central nervous system disease
   Tumor
   Head injury
   Seizure
   Infection
Drug therapy
   Corticosteroids
   Sympathomimetics
   Oral contraceptive pills
Essential

From Chapter 3, Table 3.5

Some Prescription and Nonprescription Drugs That May Cause Hypertension*

Albuterol
Amphetamines (biphetamine, dexedrine)
Amphotericin B
Antidepressants (amitriptyline, imipramine, Ativan)
Antipsychotics (Haldol)
Bromocriptine
Caffeine
Calderol
Carbamazepine (Tegretol)
Cocaine
Cyclosporine
Dexadrine
Dihydroergotamine
Dimercaprol
Ephedrine
Epinephrine
Epogen
Ethanol
Fentanyl
Gentamicin
Ketoconazole
Metaproterenol
Methylphenidate (Ritalin)
Metoclopramide HCl (Reglan)
Naphazoline HCl
Nonsteroidal anti-inflammatory drugs (ibuprofen, naproxen)
Oral contraceptives
Oxymetazoline HCl
Phenylephrine HCl
Phenylpropanolamine HCl
Promethazine HCl (Phenergan)
Pseudoephedrine HCl
Steroids (hydrocortisone, Medrol, prednisone)
Terbutaline
Tetrahydrozoline HCl
Vincristine
Xylometazoline HCl

---

*Some of the drugs listed are ingredients in many over-the-counter medications. Please refer to the package label. In addition, please refer to the Physicians Desk Reference or package inserts for potential interaction with other drugs.
From Chapter 4, Table 4.2

Evaluation of Hypertension

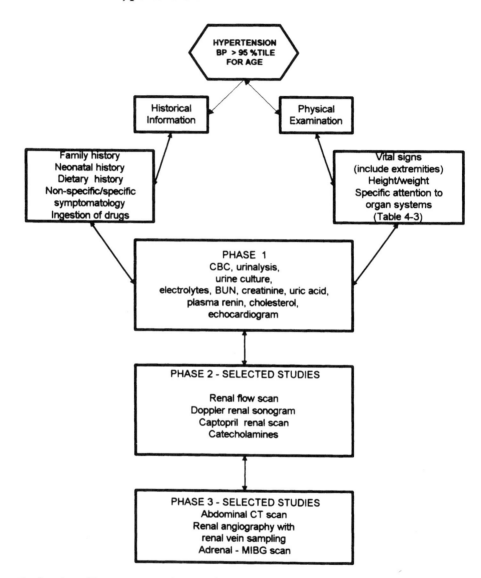

Evaluation of hypertension. (From Chapter 4, Figure 4.1)

Basic Laboratory Tests for Initial Childhood Hypertensive Evaluation

Complete blood count
Urinalysis
Urine culture
BUN, creatinine
Plasma renin activity
Uric acid
Electrolytes and total CO_2
Cholesterol and triglycerides
Echocardiogram

From Chapter 4, Table 4.4

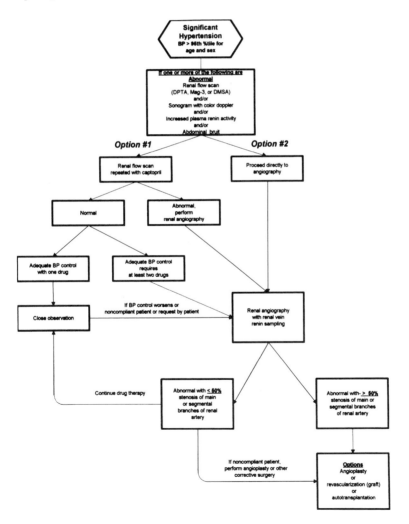

Evaluation of renovascular hypertension. (From Chapter 4, Figure 4.2)

Normal Values for Pediatric Plasma Renin Activity (PRA)

Age	Mean PRA in ng/ml/hr (range)
3 days–3 mos	12.0 (0.5–24.2)
3–12 mos	5.7 (2.2–10.2)
1–3 yrs	3.1 (0.5–8.0)
3–6 yrs	2.8 (0.1–12.0)
6–9 yrs	2.0 (0.1–7.5)
9–12 yrs	2.0 (0.2–7.0)
12–15 yrs	1.9 (0.2–8.0)
15–18 yrs	1.5 (0.2–6.5)

From Chapter 4, Table 4.5

Normal Values for Pediatric Plasma Aldosterone Levels

Age	Median in ng/dl (range)
1 wk–3 mos	62 (30–201)
3–12 mos	18 (7–39)
1–4 yrs	15 (3–77)
4–8 yrs	11 (5–20)
8–13 yrs	8 (4–17)

From Chapter 4, Table 4.11

Urinary Excretion of Vanillylmandelic Acid, Homovanillic Acid, and Total Metanephrines in Children*

Age (yrs)	Vanillylmandelic Acid		Homovanillic Acid		Total Metanephrines	
	Mean	SD	Mean	SD	Mean	SD
<1	6.9	3.2	12.9	9.6	1.6	1.3
1–2	4.6	2.2	12.6	6.3	1.7	1.1
2–5	3.9	1.7	7.6	3.6	1.2	0.8
5–10	3.3	1.4	4.7	2.7	1.1	0.8
10–15	1.9	0.8	2.5	2.4	0.6	0.5
15–18	1.3	0.6	1.0	0.6	0.2	0.2

*All values are given as milligrams per milligram of creatinine.
From Chapter 4, Table 4.9

Pharmacologic Therapy for Hypertension

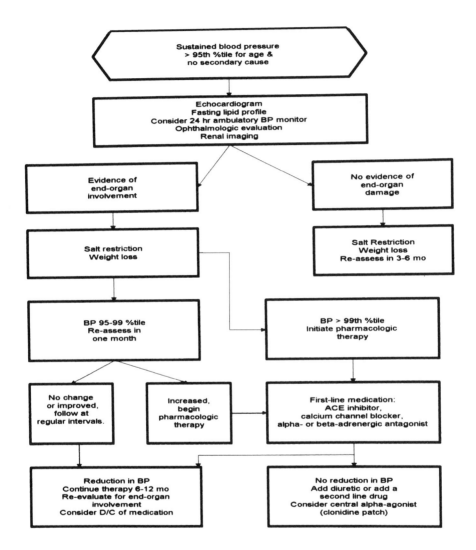

Treatment of essential hypertension in children and adolescents. (From Chapter 6, Figure 6.2)

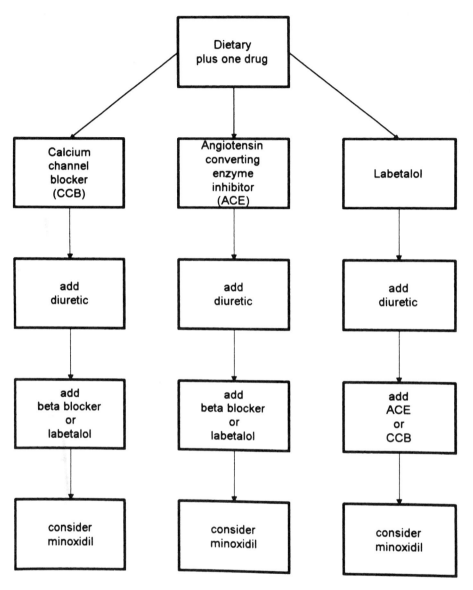

Specific treatment pathways for essential hypertension. (From Chapter 6, Figure 6.3)

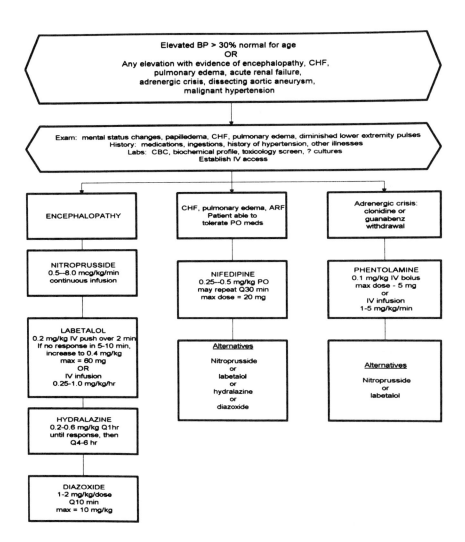

Treatment of hypertensive emergencies. (From Chapter 6, Figure 6.4)

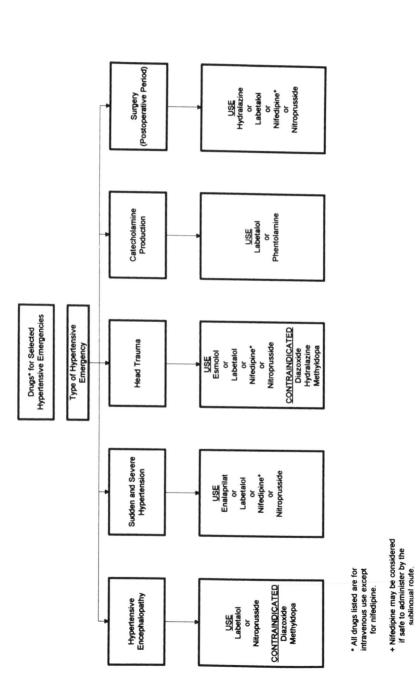

Recommended medications for specific causes of hypertensive emergencies. (From Chapter 6, Figure 6.5)

Possible Side Effects of Angiotensin-Converting Enzyme Inhibitors

Renal	Proteinuria, renal insufficiency, nephrotic syndrome (contraindicated in bilateral renal artery stenosis), hyperkalemia
Hematologic	Neutropenia, agranulocytosis, anemia, thrombocytopenia, pancytopenia
Cardiovascular	Hypotension, syncope, orthostatic hypotension
Dermatologic	Rash, angioedema, erythema multiforme
Respiratory	Cough, bronchospasm, eosinophilic pneumonitis
Gastrointestinal	Dysgeusia, pancreatitis, glossitis, dyspepsia, jaundice, hepatitis
Central nervous system	Ataxia, confusion, depression
Genitourinary	Impotence

From Chapter 6, Table 6.2

Side Effects of Calcium Channel Blockers

Common (approximately 10.0%)	Peripheral edema, dizziness, lightheadedness, nausea, headache, flushing, weakness
Less common (approximately 5.0%)	Transient hypotension
Infrequent (<2.0%)	Nasal and chest congestion, dyspnea, diarrhea, constipation, cramps, flatulence, myalgia, muscle cramps, sleep disturbances, blurred vision, rash, urticaria, sexual dysfunction
Rare (<0.5%)	Thrombocytopenia, anemia, leukopenia, allergic hepatitis, gingival hyperplasia, depression, transient blindness

From Chapter 6, Table 6.5

Side Effects of Beta Blockers

Cardiovascular effects	Bradycardia, hypotension, syncope, shock, exacerbation of angina pectoris in susceptible patients, fluid retention
Central nervous system effects	Lightheadedness, ataxia, dizziness, irritability, sleepiness, hearing loss, visual disturbances, vivid dreams/nightmares, hallucinations, weakness, fatigue, depression
Gastrointestinal effects	Nausea, vomiting, diarrhea, cramping, constipation, flatulence
Hematologic effects	Transient eosinophilia, idiosyncratic reactions of thrombocytopenia, nonthrombocytopenic purpura, agranulocytosis
Other effects	Impotence, rash

From Chapter 6, Table 6.10

Side Effects of Central Sympatholytic Drugs

Sedation
Dry mouth
Depression, vivid dreams/nightmares, hallucinations
Impotence, decreased libido, ejaculatory difficulty
Rebound hypertension when discontinued abruptly

From Chapter 6, Table 6.21

Summary of Major Side Effects of Diuretic Agents

	Loop	Thiazide	Potassium-Sparing
Hypokalemia	Yes	Yes	No
Hyperkalemia	No	No	Yes
Hypercalciuria	Yes	No	No
Hyperuricemia	Yes	Yes	No
Hypomagnesemia	Yes	Yes	No
Hyperglycemia	No	Yes	Possible
Hyperlipidemia	No	Yes	No

From Chapter 6, Table 6.13

Selected Oral Antihypertensive Dosing in Pediatrics*

Drug	Neonates	Children	Adolescent	Onset of action
Angiotensin-converting enzyme inhibitors				
Captopril	0.05–0.1 mg/kg/dose q8–12h	0.5–2.0 mg/kg/day q8h	12.5 mg q8h (max. 200 mg/day)	15 min
Enalapril	?	0.1–0.5 mg/kg/day q12–24h	2.5–40 mg/day q12–24h	30–60 min
Enalaprilat	5–10 µg/kg/dose q8–24 hrs IV	Same as neonates	1.25 mg IV q6h	5–15 min
Fosinopril	?	?	10–40 mg/day q24h	
Beta-blocking agents				
Propranolol	0.5–2.0 mg/kg/day q6–12h	0.5–2.0 mg/kg/day q6–12h (max. 8 mg/kg/day)	40 mg/dose q12h (max. 480 mg/day)	1–2 hr
Nadolol	?	?	40–160 mg q24h	
Atenolol	?	? (0.8–1.0 mg/kg/dose q24h)	50–100 mg q24h	60 min–3 hr

Drug	Neonates	Children	Adolescent	Onset of action
Metoprolol	?	?	100–200 mg q12–24h	60 min
Acebutolol	?	?	200–800 mg q24h	
Labetalol	?	? (3 mg/kg/ day q12h)	100–400 mg/day q12h	20 min–2 hr
Calcium channel–blocking drugs				
Nifedipine	0.25–2.0 mg/ kg/dose q6–8h	Same as infant	10–60 mg q8–12h (max. 180 mg/day)	10–20 min PO; 1–5 min SL
Diltiazem	?	?	60–180 mg q12h	30–60 min
Verapamil	Contraindi- cated	4–10 mg/kg/day q8h	240–480 mg/day q8–12h	80–150 min
Isradipine	?	?	2.5–5.0 mg q12h	20 min
Central sympatholytics[b]				
Clonidine	?	0.05–0.30 mg/ dose q8–12h	0.1–0.6 mg/dose q8–12h	30–60 min
Diuretics				
Chlorothia- zide	10–30 mg/kg/ day q12h	5–10 mg/kg/dose q12–24h	0.25–1.00 g/dose	
Hydrochloro- thiazide	1–3 mg/kg/day q12h	0.5–2.0 mg/kg/ dose q12–24h	25–100 mg/dose q12–24h	
Furosemide	1–4 mg/kg/dose q6–12h	0.5–2.0 mg/kg/ dose q12–24h	Same	
Bumetanide	?	?	0.5–2.0 mg/dose	
Spironolac- tone	?	1–3 mg/kg/day q12–24h	25–100 mg/day q12–24h	
Metolazone	?	0.2–0.4 mg/kg/ day q12–24h	2.5–5.0 mg/dose q12–24h	
Vasodilators				
Hydralazine	0.5–2.0 mg/kg/ dose q6h–12h IV: 0.1–0.5 mg/ kg/dose q4–6h	0.5–2 mg/kg/ dose q6–12h IV: 0.1–0.5 mg/ kg/dose q4–6h	10–50 mg/dose q6h Same	20–30 min
Minoxidil	?	0.1–0.5 mg/kg/ dose q6–12h	2.5–20 mg/dose q6–12h	30 min

? = no or limited experience; nephrology consult suggested.
*Oral dosing except as indicated.

Pharmacologic Therapy of Neonatal Hypertension

Drug	Dosing
Captopril	0.05–0.5 mg/kg/day PO divided q6–8h
Enalaprilat	5–10 μg/kg/dose q8–24h
Hydralazine	Hypertensive crisis: 0.1–0.5 μg/kg/dose IM/IV q4–6h
	Chronic hypertension: 0.5–5.0 mg/kg/day PO divided q6–12h
Chlorothiazide	20–30 mg/kg/day PO divided q12h
Hydrochlorothiazide	2–3 mg/kg/day PO divided q12h
Furosemide	1–4 mg/kg/dose IV/PO q6–8h
Propranolol	0.5–2.0 mg/kg/day PO divided q6–12h
Nitroprusside	0.5–8.0 μg/kg/min continuous IV infusion
Diazoxide	1–2 mg/kg/dose IV q10mins up to 10 mg/kg/day

From Chapter 6, Table 6.29

Selected Antihypertensive Drugs for Patients with Chronic Renal Failure

Drug	Formulation	Dose (Oral)	Adjustment in Chronic Renal Failure	Effect on Renin
Diuretics				Increase
Chlorothiazide	250- and 500-mg tablets, 250 mg/5 ml	5–10 mg/kg/ dose bid	Thiazides not effective at glomerular filtration rate (GFR)	
Hydrochloro- thiazide	25-, 50-, and 100-mg tablets, 50 mg/5 ml; 100 mg/ml	0.5–2.0 mg/ kg/dose qd or bid	<30–40 ml/ min/1.73 m^2	
Furosemide	20-, 40-, and 80-mg tablets, 10 mg/ml	0.5–4.0 mg/ kg/dose qd or bid	None	
Bumetanide	0.5-, 1-, and 2-mg tablets	0.01–0.03 mg/dose qd	Unknown	
Metolazone	2.5-, 5-, and 10-mg tablets, 0.1 mg/ml	0.2 mg/kg/ dose qd or bid	Unknown	
Beta blockers				Decrease
Acebutolol	200- and 400-mg tablets	200–800 mg qd (adults)	Decrease dose	
Atenolol	25-, 50-, and 100-mg tablets	50–100 mg (adults)	Decrease 50% at GFR <50 ml/ min/1.73 m^2, give qod GFR <10 ml/min/1.73 m^2	
Labetalol	100-, 200-, and 300-mg tablets	50–100 mg bid (>10 yrs of age)	None	
Metoprolol	50- and 100-mg tablets	100–200 mg qd or bid (adults)	None	
Propranolol	10-, 20-, 40-, 60-, and 80-mg tablets 20, 40, and 80 mg/ml	0.5–1.0 mg/ dose bid	None	
Vasodilators				Increase
Hydralazine	10-, 25-, 50-, and 100-mg tablets 0.2 mg/ml	0.5–2.0 mg/ kg/dose bid or qid	None	
Minoxidil	2.5 and 10-mg tablets	0.1–0.5 mg/ kg/dose bid to qd	None	

Selected Antihypertensive Drugs for Patients with Chronic Renal Failure *(cont.)*

Drug	Formulation	Dose (Oral)	Adjustment in Chronic Renal Failure	Effect on Renin
Central sympatholytic				Decrease
Clonidine	0.1-, 0.2-, and 0.3-mg tablets or patch	0.05–0.30 mg/ dose bid or tid	None	
Angiotensin-converting enzyme inhibitors				Increase
			Caution with all ACE inhibitors when GFR <50 ml/min/1.73 m^2	
Captopril	12.5-, 25-, 50-, and 100-mg tablets	0.5–2.0 mg/ kg/day bid		
Enalapril	2.5-. 5-, 10-, and 20-mg tablets	0.15 mg/kg/day bid		
Fosinopril	10- and 20-mg tablets	5–20 mg qd (adults)		
Lisinopril	2.5-, 5-, 10-, 20-, and 40-mg tablets	2.5–20.0 mg/day bid or qd (adults)		
Calcium channel blockers				None
Nifedipine	10- and 20-mg caplets 30-, 60-, and 90-mg sustained release	0.25–2.0 mg/ kg/dose bid to qid sustained release qd or bid	May need to limit dose	
Diltiazem	30-, 60-, 90-, 120-mg tablets 120-, 180-, 240-, and 300- mg caplets	0.40–1.25 mg/ kg/dose qid sustained release qd to bid	Unknown	
Verapamil	120-, 180-, and 240-mg tablets	4–10 mg/kg/ day tid	With caution	

From Chapter 6, Table 6.31

Index